HOW TO MAKE MILLION DOLLARS AS A SPA OWNER:

The Secret Formula to Success Revealed!

ISBN: **978-1519182876**

INTRODUCTION

Imagine a lifestyle where you can go or do anything – whenever you want. Imagine having a clientele that loves you because of everything you share with them that has helped them in so many ways. Imagine having your family time not centered around your work schedule or having to worry about money. Can this be done while still being a solo act in your profession? Absolutely.

You can attain all this, and more, with the help of this book and a simple business math formula. What's even better is that this formula guarantees your success in becoming a millionaire (provided you don't blow your money on vices or investment schemes). Every single person has the potential to become a millionaire in the next 10-12 months if they apply the principles and formula to their business, which is customized for their particular situation (solo, group, franchise, etc.).

Why aren't all people in your profession millionaires right now? This is a great question. If the formula is so easy and the fundamentals make perfect sense, then why hasn't everyone in your field figured it out? Frankly, your industry in general hasn't been geared to think or operate business in this fashion.

Never before has a formula like this been introduced to this field/industry. There's no one to blame, even though many blame instructors and schools for lack of business preparation. This is simply a new, fresh way to approach this industry's business altogether, and it works. We get so wrapped up in "service income + product income = how much we can make – expenses". That's not how we should think about business. Instead, we should be focusing on all the ways to make money using the skills, talents and digital assets we have.

Many entrepreneurs like yourself are simply conditioned to think of income in simple terms – rate multiplied by number of meetings, sessions, hours equals total income, less applicable expenses. One could add product sales in there to make it a bit more fancy but there's still a lot of opportunity for income missing.

You've probably read a lot of business books, particularly on business opportunities in your profession and generating clients and customers. You've probably left a lot of them underwhelmed by vagueness and over-simplicity. Finally, many of them have you buying a lot of marketing products like business cards, brochures, fancy websites, snake oils and products and the like. Many are marked with making a specific amount of money or becoming successful in one year or less – which are good concepts – but lack the math element that is required of a business owner to follow when attempting to generate a specific goal. So instead of spending a lot of money doing things that have no real goal in mind for a specific amount of revenue, why not spend only very little to generate a lot? Doesn't that make more sense?

The great news here is that over 75% of your business activities will be driven by your website and your limitless creativity – not by marketing gimmicks, MLMs, tiered income schemes, or affiliate links – and once set up, will draw you hundreds of thousands of dollars when followed through properly. All this, while helping clients and thousands of other people that are guaranteed to take interest in what you have to say.

Sure, there are skeptics and they're out there voicing their opinion that making becoming a millionaire in your field of expertise – especially when working for the "man" is impossible. Let them scoff and continue to follow the path of negativity if that is where they choose to reside and spend their energy. They're simply wrong in thinking that it's not possible to become a millionaire entrepreneur.

You have a choice, however. You can either take a chance on this book to improve yourself and your business for a minimal investment (a tax write-off) or you can choose not to and continue down the path you're already on, trying to figure things out along the way. It's completely up to you.

If you're ready to move beyond traditional and even "contemporary" marketing activities, then let's get started. The faster you read and comprehend this book and devise your plans to become a millionaire, the sooner it'll happen for you.

CHAPTER 1: YOU ARE A MILLIONAIRE IN THE MAKING

You are a millionaire in the making. Believe it.

The big question that everyone asks is whether or not it's possible to become a millionaire entrepreneur. Anything is possible when you become an entrepreneur. The sky is the limit, time becomes your limited resource, and you're free to create. I am living proof, and there are thousands more just like me.

Those that "get it" understand that **simply providing a service alone in the hopes of having substantial income is not enough**. You're just one person, probably with a little bit of inventory if you're like most small business owners (or maybe you're working in cube-land and are hoping to someday escape!), and have a few social media outlets that you post to from time to time. *You work your butt off and wonder, why am I not more successful by now?*

I'll tell you the answer straight out and elaborate in the rest of the chapters so you see exactly where you're missing the big picture.

You're not following a set formula that all of the other successful website owners, million-dollar bloggers and millionaire-next-door types have already figured out but never tell you.

But I'm here to blow the door wide open for you. And you don't need thousands of dollars to get going, either. I had $40 to my name when I first launched my business. And I learned from the best, just like you're learning from me now. There IS a formula that you need to follow and in Chapter 3, I'm going to tell you what it is. And after you put all of the variables into play, you're going to laugh at how easy it was (hard work, though) to follow and implement it.

There are actually several millionaires in your profession – you just wouldn't know it, and this will be explained more in Chapter 3. Think about some of the best, most highly-regarded people in your profession. Some of them have retired early, having worked hard at accomplishing their own personal goals and are financially sound enough to stop working. For some, marketing and succeeding at their business came naturally because they figured out what worked best for them. Others had to work very hard to where they got where they are in life, and are still working simply because they love what they do. And they keep raking in the money left and right.

It's a question that most millionaires hear everywhere as they tour the country on business. Will it happen for me? How did you do it? Whether it's heard in tradeshows and cities across United States or lectures given to women's and community groups, everyone wants an answer to that very question.

You don't need to be the next Bill Gates, Mark Zuckerberg or Steve Jobs to make a million dollars on the next big thing. Becoming a millionaire is not about luck or being a genius or having any special talents. You don't even have to be selling the next high-tech invention to get rich. You can do it with something as simple as diversifying your time and maximizing the profit potential with every hour you have during the day. If you've ever heard about "making money while you sleep", that's exactly what the goal is – and it's not about becoming a part of a MLM or affiliate marketing. Imagine having money pour into your business without really having to lift a finger. The secret to this is to put desired outputs "out there" that people want that they can help themselves to.

There has been no shortage of books in the last decade telling you how to think like a millionaire. Thinking like a millionaire is not enough. Books that tell you how to invest money to get rich really only work when you have money to begin with. The truth is only millionaires really understand and learn how to think like a millionaire and that is by becoming one. Many lessons are learned along the way on the path to wealth. It does not happen overnight. It does not happen simply with hard work. Becoming a millionaire requires strategy and careful planning.

This book is not just about how to become a millionaire focused on making a buck or a million of them - it's about how to become a millionaire while putting your family, employees, clients and customers first – providing immense value to your community and representing the profession for what it truly is. Being an entrepreneur - especially a wealthy one - requires a sense of ease and confidence to make everything look effortless because you are considered a leader of the "stress-free" lifestyle. You certainly will not become a millionaire while running around your shop or home office/workspace looking like a harried fanatic while trying to push sales on everyone (hint – this is SO not the way to make a million dollars). This book shows you how to go about becoming wealthy in a stress-less manner that is fun and creative.

The path is actually an easy one to take and does not require a lot of extra stress or additional work or learning that you don't already know how to do. You're just going to need these pointers contained in this book to have that one "Ah-ha" moment as you see all the pieces come together. Technology has empowered us in new and exciting ways which has a radically transforms the traditional workday of the entrepreneur, and we're going to use technology and systems to make everything work for us.

You are going to have FUN making a million dollars doing what you already love to do.

Never before has it become so possible for entrepreneurs like yourself to have it all and be financially comfortable – the schedule you so desire, the flexibility, the income and the ability to continue education and live the life you desire. Before you start delving into your big plans, however, there are a few ground rules that need to be established that will help guide you on your journey to becoming a millionaire.

Rule #1: Family comes first.

This will has always been an important one because the family is what supports us from behind the scenes. We are not in the business of marketing a lifestyle. Because of this, family still remains a big portion of our health. It's delusional to think that everything will be perfect behind the scenes while trying to make people believe in something or a concept lifestyle that is not real. Behind a lot of mommy entrepreneurs, for example, are busy moms stressed out to the max trying to put on a good front while behind the scenes they are crying from screaming children, stress, and having to lock themselves in rooms in their homes just to get work done (hiding from their own children). This is not what I believe in at all.

Millionaires in your field are very real people and they keep it that way - real. Millionaires also recognize that down time with family refuels their spirit and provides them with the comfort and confidence they need to propel them forward. If you have children at home, embrace them as part of your building process - learn from them - understand their creative methods and enjoy the crayon marks on the walls and the masses. There will be a time when you'll be able to stay at home even more to be with your children instead of racing around trying to get to work or to your next client. Family rules the heart. It's important to not lose sight of family while building wealth because if family is ignored, the family unit deteriorates while you were trying to get rich. This creates an additional distraction and heartache, making it very difficult for you to focus on important strategic steps.

Rule #2: There are no limits within set limits.

Many entrepreneurs like you have legal constrictions on how they can market themselves and what they're able to offer. It's important to realize that we need to be realistic and understand that there are limits within limits. Therefore as long as you conduct your business within the guidelines mandated by state or federal law the options that you have available to you are limitless. Keep in mind that as an entrepreneur you're still able to have other businesses and business models in the event that you should find something you enjoy doing that doesn't quite fit well within the scope of allowed practice (although this book and formula does not require you to establish any other businesses outside your ideal business). It's important to realize that you can keep to business entity separate in the event that she should have to go down that road.

Rule #3: Each and every entrepreneur has the ability and right to become a millionaire.

The fact that millionaires in your field exist is quite surprising to many. However this is mostly due to the fact that only a select few have figured out how to maximize their potential without simply focusing on number of sessions multiplied by either rate. Everything happens for reason. That is one of the most essential rules of business that millionaires have experienced on the roller coaster ride that is entrepreneurship. There will be others that read this book and eventually millionaires in the business will start popping up everywhere. How wonderful for EVERYONE involved, especially in a growing industry!

If you are a budding entrepreneur and you're looking for a book that tells you every step to turning your passion for your field into a million dollars filled with practical business advice then you have come to the right place. This is a business book full of real-life savvy business experience that many lifestyle marketers definitely do not want you to know. This book is full of inside secrets to tapping into wealth-building income, which are revealed in later chapters as fundamentals are explained and the formula addressed.

This book focuses on making you and your business extraordinarily interactive. It is simply not enough these days to put information on your website and blog. Those days are over. The select few millionaires in this industry that exist in this world have learned how to become interactive with their customers and followers 24/7. How do they make that happen you might ask? This book is going to show you how to take everything to the streets - launching your brand into a national marketplace instead of simply a local one, while enjoying a lifestyle you so rightly deserve.

- In the process you are going to get free publicity.
- You will be developing your story and the will to drive forward while assisting millions of customers all around the world
- You are going to show clients how to better their situation, their brand or their lifestyle
- You were going to become more accessible.
- You are going to become a star within your own brand.
- You are going to devise and execute an exit strategy that once you make your millions, you'll capitalize upon the sale of your company just years after start up if you so choose to exit the market.

This book is going to help you break down doors and barriers that have kept you from financial health. And, this book is going to help you focus on why actually sitting down and working on the business plan is so critical to your success.

This book focuses on a simple formula for success that sets you and your business up to make a million dollars each and every year, if not more.

However, the meaning behind each variable is significant and it is in those variables that secrets are revealed on how to make the million dollars easily possible. This book focuses on activities and revenue streams that you can start doing within 10 minutes after finishing this book. Utilizing resources and assets that you probably already have at your disposal such as a computer and camera. Sure there maybe things that you will want to buy to help you streamline your process while you follow the step-by-step instructions but those decisions are entirely up to you.

Secrets to Success

The secrets to success in becoming a million dollar entrepreneur in your profession focuses on several fundamentals which include but are not limited to time management, efficiency, education, helping others, accepting opportunities, using social media properly, having family and personal time, self-care, building your expertise and brand, creating multimedia platforms, services and products, websites, writing, establishing sales funnels, diversifying your activities, sharing and understanding your customer, and so much more.

This book discusses these fundamentals and applies the fundamentals to the formula accordingly. With 20+ chapters, you'll be able to easily refer back to sections within the book to refresh your thoughts and process the information on a continuous basis. The fundamentals are critical to your success as you approach each of the formula's activities because as an entrepreneur, you must stay true to yourself, your family, your clients, and your professional standards.

Ready to get started?

CHAPTER 2: FUNDAMENTALS & STANDING OUT IN THE CROWD

The difference between you and the millionaire in your profession right now is what they were willing to do in order to discover where they could make improvements and tailor their own business experience for themselves and their client/customers. They learned how to stand out in the crowd as the preferred person/company to buy from. They understood that not every client/customer is the ideal one.

Define Your Ideal Client/Customer

Working out who your ideal client is can happen in a variety of ways, the very best way is to decide who they are, prior to inventing a product or developing your services as this allows you to tailor your product or service specifically to meet the needs of your ideal customer. Many people still do it, the other way around, successfully; it's just more difficult to do. If you are working out who your ideal client is, ask yourself these questions:

Who do you really want to work with?

I like to work with people I like, who I can easily engage with and who share the same values as I do, it's important for you to know the type of people you want to work with. Write a description of your ideal customer and try not to leave anything out. You want this to be your perfect, ideal customer that would exist in a perfect world. Do you want to work with small business owners employing more than ten staff members? Do you want to work with stay at home moms wanting to start a small business? Do you want to work with early adopters or people that are afraid of technology? It's up to you to work out who your ideal customer is.

What problems can you solve for your ideal customer?

Once you have started to write down your ideal customer profile, ask yourself what problems can you solve for your ideal customers? Can you generate sales for them by designing a website for them? Can you teach them something to be more successful? Do you have a product that solves a problem? Do you offer a service that solves a problem? The bigger the problem you solve, the easier it is to engage your target customer and gain sales, so list their problems and list your solutions.

Where is your market located?

With online marketing it is easy to imagine your company selling products and services to the international community as a whole. This however is generally a mistake and you should narrow it down, to English speaking or Australian or American or something else more specific. Maybe you realized while doing your research that your ideal customers live in your own city, or state or maybe you realize they live in many cities around the world, but are all English speakers.

How much money do you need to earn?

To many this might seem like a strange question but it's an important determination on whether or not your chosen target customers, and the products and services you want to provide, will provide the income you need. If you're only capable of producing products or services for a finite amount of people and they will only purchase at a particular price, this becomes very important to determining your business financial viability.

How much disposable money does your ideal client earn?

If your target customers cannot afford to buy what you're selling then you'll have trouble meeting your goals. Determine in advance what type of money they can afford to spend and what type of quality of products and or services they are expecting for that amount of money and fill that need.

What types of clients do you absolutely not want to work with?

Just as important as it is to know with whom you want to work, it's potentially more important to know the types of people you absolutely do not want to work with. This doesn't mean that you are shunning them; it only means that they're not the right customers for you. Keeping the door closed to those whom aren't right for you helps you leave room for those who are and allows you to focus on those customers you want.

What types of business do your ideal clients participate in?

Do your ideal customers already have their own business, or do they work for a business? Does your ideal customer buy from your competitors? If so, why do they choose to buy from them? Knowing the activities of your ideal customer is an important way for you to get closer to them so that you can be a resource to them.

What are your core values and how will you align your business with those?

These can be very personal values and ethics, and what you want your business and brand to represent to the public. They can also be only related to your business, it's up to you. If you can match your values, and your business's values with your clients' values, you'll have a perfect match that will help you match up your marketing efforts to attract the right customers.

It's important to realize that if you work with and sell, only to people that you want to be around, like, and care about emotionally, you'll have a much better business model to work with. **You'll be able to stick with this ideal client and form a long term solid relationships**, and continue to solve their problems and fulfill their needs.

Starting Out...

Starting a business is never easy, it's a challenge for everyone no matter how much experience you have. In order to get some much needed attention in the business world, you need to think out of the box and find a way to set your business apart from your competition, in other words you want to stand out and be remembered for all the right things. There are a few things you can do to achieve this, and we're going to take a look at some ideas that will help people identify your brand.

Know Your Target Audience

First and foremost you have to know who your audience is. You don't want to be selling car parts to someone that's looking for gardening supplies. Identify your audience. What are they looking for? What do they need? What other things besides what you're offering are they interested in? In fact, imagine just one person your ideal customer and find out every single thing you can about them. Then all you need do is speak to this person, because it's rare for a business to be in tune with the needs of their audience nowadays and by targeting your brand to meet the needs of your target audience, your brand will automatically stand out more and engage better.

Build a Presence in Your Community

So much emphasis has been put on internet marketing recently that businesses often forget to follow through with conventional marketing. A great way to set yourself apart from the rest is to get involved in your community. Make a donation to a local charity. Join the local chamber of commerce and other business associations, many will give you their membership list simply by joining and attending events helps get you known in the local community. Small businesses need a dedicated local following and the best way to build that up is to get involved with your community.

Build a Presence on Social Media

The online presence of your business will always be important when it comes to building your brand. Be interactive, get people involved. Don't limit yourself to certain social media sites, you need to be using all of them. That means Facebook, Twitter, Linkedin, Tumblr, Pinterest, Google Plus and any other social network you can think of. The more fan pages you create, the better the chances are that someone will find you, although I have to be honest and say I'm a Twitter addict, in my opinion it's the best and I often refer to it as a global telephone directory, allowing me to make contact with almost anyone.

Create a Unique Website

Social media presence is a must but a lot of businesses sacrifice a presence on their own website in order to keep up with their social networks. Don't do that, your website is the digital equivalent of a business card and you don't want to neglect it, in facts it's most likely the most important marketing tool you can have. Create or hire someone to create a website which is unique and interactive. Social media is a great way to get people involved but your website should be a direct portal to your business.

Write a Press Release

A press release is something so simple that could help you see big results. Putting out a press release about your newest product or service and distributing it to local newspapers and other forms of media can build hype and get you attention. This is your chance to talk up your business and get some eyes on what you're doing.

I've had great success with press releases, I've had half page articles written about me, had my photograph taken numerous times, been featured in various business newspapers and all as a result of press releases.

Use Video Marketing

Commercials are a classic form of advertising but they can get expensive. A modern alternative to a TV commercial which is often overlooked is video marketing through a platform such as YouTube. You can film a commercial or other type of promotional video for little money and reach thousands of people by promoting it online.

When it comes to marketing your business, the sky is the limit. Don't make the same mistakes that others do. Make sure you distinguish your business by covering all aspects of marketing, both conventional and unconventional. Give these a try and don't be afraid to experiment.

Advertising on a Budget

You've no doubt heard about businesses generating leads, sales and new customers online and chances are you've always associated these businesses with having large online marketing budgets. You however live in the real world and you don't have the budget needed to compete online. It is however possible for you to market your business online inexpensively, I know I do it, constantly.

You can market your business for almost free if you know what to do. This is why online marketing is so much fun, because the smallest of companies can to some extend complete with the largest. The barrier to entry is low, and even the learning curve is relatively small which means that you, and anyone else can market your business effectively online with no real budget whatsoever.

Content Marketing

Content marketing should form the backbone of all your online marketing efforts, it's the single most effective form of online marketing you can do. It also provides much of the content you need for types of marketing including every single inexpensive way we are discussing today. Content is needed that educates, engages, informs, excites and ultimate that sells. You need content for all aspects of marketing, up to and including customer service.

Social Media

Social media like Twitter, LinkedIn, Facebook, Pinterest and Google+ all have a place in your online marketing efforts. One of the biggest mistakes I see is businesses trying to be the best they can be on all social media channels, unless you have lots of staff that can devote lots of time to social media you are much better to do one or two social media platforms well, than three or more poorly.

You have to try and determine which social media networks work for you, what are you passionate about? It also depends on your niche and your audience. Where do they hang out? Be there. Let me put neck on the line and say that you should be on Twitter, in my opinion every single business should be active on Twitter, it generates much more website traffic and audience engagement than any other social media platform.

Blog Often

Every single business website should incorporate a blog, it shouldn't be an external link to an external blogging platform it should actually be part of your website. Blogging regularly is a great source of website traffic, and in many instances this is the only source of traffic.

Blogging not only attracts traffic, it is also a great way to get your message out to your audience, building your authority in their eyes, while you are not spending much money on it. You can write the posts yourself or you can outsource. Most people write them themselves when starting out. It can take time to get used to doing it, but writing a post a day can help you gain momentum, but it's a long term game, so don't expect instant results.

Search Engine Optimization

If you are not familiar with SEO (search engine optimization), it's important to learn. SEO changes constantly and is how you optimize your website for search engines. If you combine basic SEO techniques with content marketing / blogging than your website will start to generate much better SEO results.

Send Out a Press Release

The good, old-fashioned press release is still exists, believe it or not and better still it continues to work. You can get a lot of value out of sending out free press releases if you know how to do it. The trick is to have contacts to which you can send the press release in hand, and better still to have engaged them previous and understand how your press release can meet their own needs.

Newsletter

Unless you have an irresistible product or service and I've yet to see one, the chances of selling to someone on their first visit to your website is slim to impossible. This means you should try to build your email subscription list, because once someone is on it, you have the chance to convert them to customers over a much longer period. This is why you need a newsletter, unless you have a large subscription base you can run your newsletter from your website with little or no additional costs.

Perfect Your Website

Your website is your store front, and even if you have a bricks and mortar store front, your website is the store front your customers will almost certainly see first. If it doesn't look great, why would anyone purchase from you? And if you expect people to find you, having a static website that is never updated isn't going to work, incorporate that blog and post something regularly if you want visitors to your website.

Get Involved In Relevant Communities

Online communities are a great way to get your name out there and to be seen in the right company. There are communities you can join on Facebook and LinkedIn, as well as self-hosted and owned "inner circles" and mastermind clubs that you can join. They can help you get known as an expert, as well as help you get more links to your website. You can also join communities with your competitors and share and learn from one another, I've found this extremely useful and of great benefit.

Finding inexpensive ways to market your business online is a great way to help you get started. But even if you have a great business, you'll want to keep using these inexpensive ways to market your business, simply because they are so effective. As you can see, much of it forms the basis of content marketing, with the content you create being used across multiple marketing channels to maximize results.

Increase Traffic to Your Website

Many people mistakenly believe that the more website visitors they attract the more sales and leads they will generate, based on the misconception that more visitors equals more sales. Whereas what you actually need are more of your target audience to visit if you want to make more sales. If you haven't already you might want to read this article on how to define your ideal client. Now that we understand the importance of attracting the right audience let's look at seven cost effective ways to increase traffic to your website.

Social Media Selling

Social media selling is free, it does however cost time and energy. The beautiful thing about social media is that it's all about interacting with others and that's exactly how you drive traffic to your website. Whether you're using Facebook, Twitter, LinkedIn or another social media platform, they key ingredient to success is interaction. Create a complete and compelling profile, interact, share and comment on items your target audience are interested in. Then when it's appropriate, post links to your website and your website content, these simple actions will drive visitors to your website and the more you interact with your target audience the more of these will visit. I'm a big fan of Twitter for driving traffic to websites and my own Twitter account drives in excess of five thousand visitors to my own website each month, with some work you could do likewise.

Comment on industry niche blogs and forums

It's amazing how much website traffic regular blog comments can generate. Simply locate some industry specific blogs your target audience frequent, subscribe and then when appropriate and when your comments are relevant, leave a comment on a new blog post. Ensure you register with the website and complete your profile fully including the website URL, as people can then click on your profile and visit your website. By getting involved, fellow commenters, forum members and blog readers are sure to visit your website on occasion. The secret is to make sure your comments represent you and your business effectively.

Blogging and Content Marketing

Every business needs a blog and this blog needs to be situated on its main website. By understanding your target audiences problems, concerns and worries and then addressing these in your blog and in particular how your products and services solve these problems. You will not only attract an audience to you, you will attract an audience wanting your products and services.

It's also extremely beneficial to guest blog on select websites that attract your target audience. Allowing guest blogging and actually guest blogging expands your reach and more importantly your areas of influence.

Publishing

Publishing remains one of the best ways to drive visitors to your website, simply gather together a selection of relevant blog posts and repackage them as an eBook or expand upon them and create an eReport. By distributing this on social media, to your friends and by allowing those that download it to freely distribute it to their friends and associates you can reach new potential customers.

Advertising Campaigns

You can make money by advertising or you can lose a lot of money advertising. If you understand who your audience is and are tightly focussed on reaching only these and manage your campaign strategically it can be very cost effective. The secret is to remain focused on your target customers and to send people to a specific page. For example, send them to a dedicated sales page, landing page or opt-in page, by doing so you can track the results and keep control of your budget.

Affiliate Program

Starting an affiliate program is a big undertaking and can a fair amount of time, but it doesn't have to cost the earth. A well-managed and well support affiliate network can send a lot of website traffic your way and you only pay for results, think of your affricates as commission only sales people. It's an extremely cost effective and rewarding way to generate business I know, in the early zeros I had over three thousand affiliates marketing my products. The secret is to have a product that appeals to both your target audience and affiliates, if your affiliates like it, understand it and can see a way to market it easily you can succeed with this.

Generating website traffic doesn't have to cost the earth, all you need do is work out your goals and then plan to achieve them using whatever budget you have, if any. Track, Modify and repeat for success, it really is as simple as that. One final tip is to do what you are comfortable doing, I personally spend my time blogging and content marketing, social media selling (as it seems to be called now) and this generates over 500,000 page views per month … and costs just my time, you could potentially improve upon this.

Review of the Fundamentals

Let's review the fundamentals again. Time management, efficiency, education, helping others, accepting opportunities, using social media properly, having family and personal time, self-care, building your expertise and brand, creating multimedia platforms, services and products, websites, writing, establishing sales funnels, diversifying your activities, sharing and understanding your customer, etc. Marketing is a big part of all of these fundamentals, especially a special kind of marketing – word of mouth.

Everything begins and ends with you. Then, everything begins and ends with your website. It's the one piece of real estate you cannot live or function without. This is the one key area of your marketing platform that

you need to spend time and money on. Hire a designer if you have to —
make it appealing, easy to use and attractive.

CHAPTER 3: THE MILLIONAIRE LIFESTYLE, THE CODE, AND ENTREPRENEURSHIP – USING THE SECRET FORMULA TO SUCCESS

The Millionaire Code

There is a certain code that millionaires live by, particularly the quiet ones that live next door that you'd never know where millionaires in the first place. They do not flaunt their lifestyle. They make careful purchasing decisions, yet will occasionally splurge because they feel they are deserving of a reward. They take care of their children first and then the nonprofits. They give carefully, selectively choosing where their attention is most merited. They ignore trivial multi-level marketing organizations, referral business organizations with sales pitches and fees, and have no need to join the newest craze of get-rich-quick wraps, supplements and snake oils.

They're quiet about their success. As a millionaire, there's an expectation that you will follow this "code", if you will, once you attain that level. Quietly celebrated success is classy. Some millionaires in your profession are not as classy – some had family money that attributed to their success, others inherited it. Many millionaires came about their lifestyle in unscrupulous ways. I'm going to show you how to make a fortune while staying classy.

That being said, the millionaire lifestyle is not without having a lot of benefits. I have a lot of fun with money. Money makes things a lot easier when you have it. It's not so much fun when you don't. And believe me, there were times I did not have a dime to my name when I was in college. I'm sure you've had moments in your own life that you wish there had been more money. Or even a credit card with a $300 limit on it just to get you by.

Now, I'm able to donate money to charitable causes and even fulfill a charity's entire financial need for the year. I enjoy going to galas, balls and events and donating money to causes like children's care, March of Dimes and helping the local pet shelter with their financial needs. This is something that is extremely important to me. What is important to you? Write it down right now.

In addition, my private life and family finances have dramatically improve, as well. Our house is completely paid for. Our children have their college educations ready to be paid for in trusts. We have a cabin in northern California that we enjoy going to on the weekends, and now have a yacht that we take out for a week or two when we need to get away from all the hustle and bustle of "traditional" life. And yes, if you're wondering, we have to employ a captain to run it for us because of its size, and, well, we haven't earned a captain's license yet in order to navigate the ocean waters for a long journey. These are the things that I would have never dreamed about being able to do 20 years ago.

I Was Just Like You a Few Years Ago

I bumped into a guy the other day at the local coffee shop around the corner from my old office and was talking to him about what I do and such. I remember when I was first starting out, and having to exercise my elevator pitch for 30 seconds at a time. Oh, goodness.

When I told him what I do now (travel nonstop and photography with my husband, mostly, and some website work every now and then) and what I used to do, he was intrigued.

"How did you get to where you are now – you don't have to work?" he asked.

"Actually, no. I'm 42 now and am enjoying life and only work when it looks like a fun project to be a part of," I told him.

"Hmmmm," he said, contemplating my response. He was dressed in an expensive suit and tie and reminded me much of an investment banker of some sort. Probably works on commission for some brokerage firm or something, advising people what to do with their money. Not that there's anything wrong with that. But gosh, if I were him, I'd be telling everyone about this formula that I nailed down and implemented into a small business setting on how to *make money* instead of how to save it and invest it.

We talked about what he did and he pulled the standard elevator speech trick and handed me his business card. I stuffed it in my purse. He turned with his coffee in hand and walked out the door in a hurry, probably to get to his next appointment. Turns out, he was an accountant in a small firm. He was a partner and was willing to do my next tax return. I almost felt bad for the guy. He's exactly the type of person this book is for – the hard-working people that are great at what they do and spend their life doing elevator pitches, attending networking meetings and underbidding jobs just to get clients, only to raise their fees the following year and end up losing them to the other accountant down the street. And he'd have to do it all over again to replace that client with a new one. All because he hadn't figured out the key concepts of the millionaire business formula.

I *did* feel bad for him, actually. It doesn't have to BE that way. What if I told you I could help you make all the business come to you just by using a computer? Before you think I'm not a humble person, let's talk about what happened next.

As I drank my cappuccino, I thought back to my start in small business. Gosh, those were the days. I remember not eating hardly anything other than spaghetti and ramen noodles for a week because my rent for my space was due on the same day as my apartment lease. I was happy working 80 hours instead of 40 just so I didn't have to report to some senior vice president. I would do anything and everything just not to have to work that horrible job again. I couldn't be contained in a cube. *Things had to change. Fast.*

I read book after book about how to manage a small business, become a successful blogger, work my way up the corporate ladder – everything. I even tried MLM businesses that always failed because I was usually part of the last fleet to join before the MLM got boring and was replaced with the next best thing. I spent thousands on attending seminars learning about running a business from home, only to be presented with additional products that cost another few thousands of dollars in order to find out the true "secret".

Sound familiar? Well, it ends today, now that you have this book. I've earned my success, have documented exactly how I got there, and am now sharing it with you. You deserve the same things I have, and it's my belief that all people on the planet can work their way towards owning whatever they want to have and send their kids to college debt-free.

These are things that are attainable when you're smart with your choices. I could have given up and went back to working a corporate job like some hopeless droid. But no – I stuck it out, read a lot, learned a lot, followed a lot of people and here I am today, teaching you everything I know.

You May Become a Leader – Be Prepared

There are some common traits found in successful entrepreneurs and business leaders. You most likely have some of these traits already and those you don't can be developed if it's a goal of yours to become a successful business leader. Oh, and remember you don't have to lead an army of employees to reap the benefits of learning these skills. If you choose to employ people these are good to know. Even if you're just working with independent contractors or freelancers you're going to need to take time to hone in on these skills and traits.

The top seven traits of a successful business leader include:

Business Leaders Know When to Delegate Tasks.

An important skill for any entrepreneur or business leader to learn is the art of delegation, delegating to others means that you must identify the strengths and weaknesses of those on your team and capitalize on the strengths by passing out tasks accordingly.

Maintain a Positive Attitude.

Keeping your team upbeat and optimistic means that you must maintain a positive attitude and present an energetic front to your team. There must be productivity to meet goals, but you should be able to balance the working hours with some fun times. When those around you see your positive attitude, it becomes contagious and will affect your whole team.

Ethical and Honest.

Always hold yourself and those who work with you to a high level of honesty and ethics and never sacrifice this, no matter what the short term gain might be. Your team, associates and followers are reflections of you, so if you practice honest and ethical behavior, they will follow your pattern.

Ability to Communicate.

Ronald Reagan was well known as "The Great Communicator," and looking back at his lifestyle, it's easy to understand why. He was able to clearly explain and focus on what needed to be done and express it in a way that was easily understood. If you have trouble communicating, read books, study or take a course in better communication skills.

Ability to Commit.

George Patton, a well-known general in World War II was a soldier who got up close and personal to those under his command. He fought in the trenches and made it a point to be wherever his men were experiencing difficulty. As a leader, you must make a commitment to lead by example.

Maintain a Sense of Humor.

The day to day activities of being a leader can wear you down if you are not careful. If however you maintain a sense of humor through the discouraging times, your team will continue to maintain a high moral and be more effective.

Creativity.

A real leader should have the ability to change from a path they're on to another path by taking a creative stance. Sometimes, the decision involves how you're guiding others, but whatever the reason, creativity helps everyone work towards the goal you're seeking to achieve.

You need to become a true leader of yourself if you want to accomplish great things or achieve small goals. Leading your team through trials and tribulations is another reason to know how to lead. If your aspiration is to become the best business leader of your own company, or the best entrepreneur it's vitally important that you know how to lead.

The Millionaire Formula

So here's the formula that you need to follow. It's simple, but long. And it's going to serve you for years to come.

Services + Products + Employee income + eBooks + Videos + Freelancing + Coaching + Training + Consulting + Speaking + Events + Design + Donations + Courses + Audio + Webinars + Reports + Books + Branded Merchandise + DVDs + Syndication + Creative Apps + Advertising Income + Affiliate Marketing + Selling/Flipping of Intangible Assets = $1,000,000

You're probably sitting there, overwhelmed, thinking, whoa. That's a lot of variables on one side of the equation. Some of you are thinking… impossible. The rest of you are set to go, thinking – okay – how much of each equals $1,000,000? And how fast can I make it?

That's where this formula is so BEAUTIFUL It's completely up to you! But let's just go through a scenario.

Let's say you do $50,000 in services each year. You sell $5,000 in product every month. And that's where it stops. You're making $110,000 a year, right? And then you have expenses and such which cut into that number. Well, what if you were to add income off of employees or contractors you hire, eBook revenue, revenue from videos, freelancing income, coaching income, training money, consulting fees, speaking engagement fees, royalties from your designs and methods, donations to your site, money from your courses, audio royalties, webinar class fee income, report income, book income, branded merchandise income, DVD royalty income, syndication (podcasting and such) income, creative apps and software downloads income, advertising income from renting out your website, affiliate marketing income (where people click on links to buy stuff on other sites from your website) and income from you selling or flipping other sites that you build?

Do you have any idea how much that could amount to? It's crazy, right? That's an insane amount of extra untapped revenue that could be yours – but you're leaving it for someone else to have.

Let's change the amounts and I'll put it in order with the formula above:

$50,000 (Services) + $60,000 (Products) + $150,000 (Employee income) + $100,000 (eBooks) + $130,000 (Videos) + $25,000 (Freelancing)+ $50,000 (Coaching) + $25,000 (Training) + $150,000 (Consulting)+ $20,000 (Speaking) + $50,000 (Events) + $5,000 (Design) + Donations ($1,000) + $50,000 (Courses) + $25,000 (Audio) + $25,000 (Webinars) + $25,000 (Reports) + $10,000 (Books) + $10,000 (Branded Merchandise) + DVDs ($15,000) + $5,000 (Syndication) + $5,000 (Creative Apps & Software) + $5,000 (Advertising Income) + $5,000 (Affiliate Marketing) + $4,000 (Selling/Flipping Intangible Assets) = $1,000,000.

Okay, you're thinking. That's a lot of income from other stuff besides my basic services and products. You're right. It is. And it's all income and ancillary activities that you can set up to make income for you overnight while you sleep. Somewhere in Australia – on the other side of the world, another person in your profession is looking at your website and wants to know what's in your eBook. They buy it. And it's 3:23 a.m. where you are, and you're fast asleep. They happily pay $10 or $20 for what you've written. You wake up the next morning and find money and a new order having been fulfilled. Amazing, isn't it?

And you laugh because you still haven't left your "real job" in the cube or at the business you're currently at. Or maybe you laugh because everything you learned here is actually working. Because it does if you do it right.

Speaking of which… did I mention that I'm going to tell you exactly what you need to do and give you tips in the process? Good… just wanted to make sure we're on the same page.

What if you don't want to have employees – ever? Then take them out of the equation. Make up that income somewhere else. That means you might have to sell more eBooks to make up the difference. Or offer an extra class to make the same amount of money. The formula is flexible, really. You get to dictate how much revenue should be allocated where. Wonderful, right?

How will you know how much revenue should be generated from which angles? It really depends on you and what you're most comfortable in. If you're a great writer and have a knack for design, or are willing to pay people to do it for you for a fantastic downloadable product, then do a lot of revenue with eBooks. If you like being on video then your channels of choice are probably DVDs, online videos, webinars, and YouTube. This is totally up to you! You're in control.

Bottom line, that's the formula. You have a ton of options to bring in money that is relevant to your profession and applicable to an audience that puts value on your education and experience. The next trick is, setting up the platform and getting people to visit all your channels. That's where the fundamentals of the secret millionaire formula come into play.

CHAPTER 4: HOW MILLIONAIRES VIEW & VALUE TIME MANAGEMENT – TIPS FROM THE TOP

If you're reading this book, you're probably very committed to your business idea. In fact, it may even be your full-time job now. Some of you have quit your jobs to live the life of a writer, and others are still working another job to support themselves enough to be an author fulltime. And then there are those that have no intention of quitting their career – they're just looking for additional income or success as a writer on the side. Whatever group you fall under, know that this book treats your chosen business idea as a career choice – an undertaking that demands commitment and dedication – and that whatever group you fall under, there's help for you here to succeed.

Given that, the issue of time management needs to be addressed. Some of you have the whole day to write. Others have just a couple of hours a week. Time is valuable regardless of how much time you can allocate to your business. So to try to understand productivity and get the most out of it, we need to compartmentalize things a bit.

A written list of things to do is a simple technique that can increase your productivity by 20% or more, if you don't use it already. It also has extra benefits of clearing your mind and saving you energy and stress. Try to spend 5 to 10 minutes each day planning your activities with a daily to-do list. Start your day with it. Even better, every evening create your plan for the next day, listing your daily things to do. It is important that you actually write your list down – don't just mentally prepare it.

Some people are more comfortable doing it on paper, while others like to type everything up. Try and see which works better for you. To be more efficient with your time, though, use Dragon Dictation or OmniFocus.

These are great apps to get your thoughts down quickly and do not involve a pen and paper.

After you identify all your tasks, review your to-do list, evaluating on the priority of each task. Give higher priority to the tasks that gets you closer to your goals. This will help you get set for the day so you can focus on your business while getting other tasks completed as well.

Technique to Prioritizing

A principal technique is an ABC rating of your priorities. Rate your to-do list with A's if they are critical for your goals and simply must be done that day or else you face serious consequences. B's are less urgent but still important tasks that can be done once you're done with A's. C's are nice things to do that you could do if you have any time left over after A's and B's. Those tasks can be moved safely to another day.

One thing important to keep in mind – if during the day some new unplanned task comes up, don't do anything until you put the new task on your list and rate it by priority. See it written among other tasks and put it in perspective. The more you let go of the urge to skip other tasks and rush to the next most urgent matter, the more productive and satisfied you will become.

When making a to-do list, break down your complex tasks into smaller manageable pieces, and focus on one at a time.

Finally, after completion of a task, take a moment to look at the results and feel the satisfaction of the progress. We're going to use this feeling of associated success with a small task completion to condition you into working your business productively.

Decision Making

We use our decision-making skills to solve problems by selecting one course of action from several possible alternatives. Decision-making skills are also key component of time-management skills.

Decision-making can be hard. Almost any decision about some conflict can be a distraction. The difficult part is to pick one solution where the positive outcome can always avoid losses. Avoiding decisions often seems easier. Yet, making your own decisions and accepting consequences is the only way to taking control of your time, your success, and your life. If you want to learn more on how to make a decision, here are some decision-making tips to get you started.

A significant part of decision-making skills is in knowing and practicing good decision-making techniques. One of the most practical decision-making techniques can be summarizing those simple decision-making steps:

- Identify the purpose of your decision. What is the problem to be solved? Why should it be solved?
- Get information. What factors does it include?
- Identify the principles to judge the alternatives. What standards and judgment criteria should the solution meet?
- Possible choices that lead to solutions.
- Evaluate each choice in terms of its consequences. Use your standards and judgment criteria to determine the cons and pros of each alternative.
- Determine the best alternative. This is much easier after you go through the above preparation steps.
- Put the decision into action. Move your decision into a specific plan of action steps. Next make a plan.
- Evaluate the outcome of your decision and action steps. What lessons can be learned? This is important stuff for the development of your decision-making skills and judgment.

Here's one final remark on decision making. In everyday life we often have to make decisions fast, without enough time to systematically go through the above actions and thinking steps. Evaluate each situation and identify the most effective decision-making strategies to keep an eye on your goals and then let your intuition suggest you the right choice.

The Issue of Time

Perhaps the greatest single problem that people have today is time property – who or what your time should belong to at any given point. Working people have too much to do in the little time they have in their personal lives. Most people feel overwhelmed with responsibilities and activities. The sense of being on a never-ending treadmill can cause you to fall into the reactive/responsive mode of living.

This is clearly a conflict of deciding what you want to do, so you can generally react to what is happening around you. Pretty soon you lose all sense of control. You feel that your life is running you, rather than you running your life. Basically, you have to stand back and take stock of yourself and what you're doing. You have to stop the clock and do some serious thinking about who you are and where you're going. You have to evaluate your activities in the light of what is really important to you. You must master your time rather than becoming a slave to the constant flow of events and demand anytime. And you must organize your life to achieve balance, harmony, and inner peace. Because if you don't, instead of running your business a book fast you're going to be frustrated and grasping at straws as to what to do next with your time.

Taking action without thinking, especially in business, is the cost for every failure. Your ability to think is the one true trade skill that you possess. If you improve the quality of your thinking, you can improve the quality of your life and business, sometimes immediately. Time is the most precious resource. It is the type of thing you have only so much of. It is perishable, it is irreplaceable, and it cannot be saved. It can only be reallocated from a task of lower value to activities of higher value.

Our work in the service and product business requires time. And time is actually essential for the important relationships in your life. The very act of taking a moment to think about your time before you spend it will begin to improve your personal time management immediately. I used to think that time management was only business tool, like a calculator or cellular telephone. It was something that you used so that you could get more done in a short period of time. I thought time management could be used exclusively to make more money in a shorter period of time.

Then I learned that time management is not a preferred activity or skill. It is a core skill upon which everything else in life depends. In your work or business life there are many demands on your time for other people. Very little of your time is yours to use as you choose. However, at home and in your personal life you can seek management of control over how you use your time.

And it is in this area that I want to focus. Personal time management begins with you – especially when you want to use your time as a writer. It begins with your thinking through what is really important to you in life. And it only makes sense if you organize it around specific goals that you want to accomplish.

You need to set goals in the three major areas of your life. First you need family and personal goals. These are the reasons why you get up in the morning, why you work hard and upgrade your skills, and why you worry about money. What are your personal and family goals, both tangible and intangible? A family goal could be a bigger house, a better car, larger television set, vacation, or anything else that costs money and an intangible goal would be to build your quality relationship with your spouse and children, to spend more time with your family going for walks and reading books. Even the family personal goals are the real essence of time management, and its major purpose.

The second area of goals is your business and career goals. These are the money goals, the means by which you achieve your personal, the why goals. How can you achieve the level of income that will enable you to the field of your family goals? How can you develop the skills and abilities to stay ahead of the curve in your career? Business and career goals are actually central ones, especially when balance with family and personal goals.

The third type of goals is your personal about-me goals. Remember, you can't achieve much more on the outside if you haven't achieved much inside. Your outer life will be a reflection of your inner life. If you wish to achieve worthwhile things in your personal and your career life, you must become a worthwhile person in your own self-development. You must build yourself if you want to build your life. Perhaps the greatest success secret is that you can become anything you really want to become to achieve any goal that you really want to achieve. But in order to do it, you must go to work on yourself, your business, and never stop.

Once you have a list of your personal goals, your author business goals, and your self-improvement goals, you can then organize the list by priority. This brings us to the difference between priority and posterior goals. In order to get your personal life under control, you must decide very clearly upon your priorities. You must decide on the most important things that you could possibly be doing to give yourself the same amount of happiness, same action, to be enjoying your life.

But the same time, you must establish posterior goals as well. Just as priorities are things that you could do more of as evidence you are, posterior goals are things that you can do less of and at a later time.

The fact is, your calendar is full. You have no spare time. Your time is extremely valuable. Therefore, for you to do anything new, you will have to stop doing something old. In order to get into something, you will have to get out of something else. In order to pick something up, you'll have to put something down. Before you make any new commitment of your time, you must really decide what activities you're going to discontinue any personal life. If you want to spend more time with your family, for example, you must decide what activities you currently engage in that are preventing you from doing so.

Principal time management says that hard time pushes out of time. This means that hard time such as working pushes out some time, such as the time you spend with your family. If you don't get your work done at the office because you don't need your time all, you must invariably have to rob that time from your family.

As a result, because your family is important to you, you find yourself in a values conflict. You feel stressed and irritable. You feel tremendous amount of pressure. You know in your heart that you should be spending more time with those people in your life, but because you didn't get your work done, you have to fulfill those responsibilities before you can spend time with your spouse and children. Your business suffers because of the guilt you feel. Then when you actually are granted some time to write, you've lost every great idea you had – because you were too slow in getting everything down, and didn't write as you go along.

They get it. Every minute you waste in the waking hours of the daytime your family could have ultimately beautified. Concentrate on working when you're at work so that you can concentrate on your family when you're at home. Concentrate on working quickly with your business so that you can earn more money to have even MORE time with your family (as in, being able to write whenever you want and not have to work for "the man").

There are three key questions that you can ask yourself continually to give your personal life and your business some balance. The first question is "what is really important to me?" Whenever you find yourself asking what you must do in so little time, stop and ask yourself, "what is it that is so important for me to do in this situation?" Then make sure you are doing is the answer to that question.

The second question is, "what are the highest value activities?" In your personal life, this means, "what are the things that I can do that give me the greatest pleasure and most action?" Or, "Of all the things that I could be doing at any one time, what are the things that I could do to add the greatest value to my life?"

And the final question for you to ask over and over again is "what is the most valuable use of my time right now?" Since you can only do one thing at a time you need to organize your life so that you're doing one thing, the most important thing, at every moment. **Personal time management enables you to choose what to do first, what did you second, and what not to do it all.** It enables you to organize every aspect of your life so that you can get the greatest joy, happiness, and achievement out of everything you do.

What is the point of time management? Time management takes time and effort, and it is always much easier when you have a simple system of practical roles and hints that are easy to keep in mind. That is exactly what the tips below are for.

- Know what you want from me time.
- Set goals into something smart that makes sense.
- Learn the difference between urgent and important.

The important tasks are those that lead you to your goals, and give you the most of your long-term progress and reward. Those tasks are very often not urgent. Many urgent tasks are not really important.

Know and Respect Your Priorities

Remember to do the important things first. Remember the 80/20 rule: 80% of reward comes from 20% of effort. One of the aims of time management is to help you refocus your mind and give more attention and time to those most important 20%.

- Find directions for achieving your goals. Plan your actions for achieving your goals
- Convert your goals into the system a specific actions to be done.

The first significant point of planning is the planning process itself. It is a known fact, and you will see it for yourself, that the planning process stimulates your brain to come up with new efficient solutions. It programs your subconscious mind to search for some shortcuts. It makes you much more prepared for each specific action. Besides, planning will help you identify potential competent crises, minimizing the number of urgent tasks. And it does amazing things for your outline and writing processes!

Planning can also significantly lower the time spent on routine maintenance tasks. Also remember that planning and related time management tips work best when you preview your plans regularly.

A Concentration Test

Your concentration can be easily lost in the sea of many boring and less important things waiting to be done in your head. Things circulating in your mind are also a big drain of your mental energy. Most often, there is no way to get those things out of your mind except of either doing them or scheduling them in a trustful system, and convincing your mind that they will be done and your time.

Know How You Spend Your Time

Keep a time log timeframe usage in 15 min. intervals, or like a week, and then analyze it to see where your time goes. For example, what percentage of time do you spend on urgent and on important activities, and what you dedicate your most time to. You are likely to be surprised, and you will see much better if you could use it for better time management. This is also an effective way to get feedback on how well these time management tips and techniques are working for you, and where you need some adjustments.

Time management skills are your abilities to recognize and solve personal time management problems. The goal of these time skills is to show you what you can do to improve the skills you've learned and apply them.

With good time management skills you are in control of your time in your life, of your stress and energy levels. You make progress at work and in your writing. You are able to maintain balance between your work, personal, and family lives. You have enough flexibility to respond to surprises or new opportunities.

All time management skills are learnable. Most likely you'll see much improvement from simply becoming aware of the essence and causes of common personal time management problems. With these time management lessons, you can see better which time management techniques are most relevant for your situation. Many of your problems, including the blank screen syndrome, will gradually disappear.

Here's the beauty of the situation. You already know how you should be managing your time, so please hold onto it, and don't give up. What you may be overlooking is the psychological side of your time management skills; psychological obstacles hidden behind your personality.

Depending on your personal situation, things such as school or work may be the primary reason why you procrastinate, have difficulty saying no, delegating, or making time management decisions. The psychological component of your time management skills can also be dealt with.

The major bottleneck in any planning or problem-solving process is brainstorming or generating new ideas and options versus specific actions and solutions.

The resulting outcome of your solution or plan is only as good as your best options and ideas you put in it. It is also important how fast you can come up with new ideas, as you will need many of them in your time management and decision-making.

Fortunately, there are ways to significantly improve your effectiveness in brainstorming your ideas. Though sometimes we're brainstorming with first-degree brainstorming sessions, here we look at how you can bring some to generate ideas on your own.

With very few exceptions, everyone already has a natural ability of creative thinking. Yet, the creative ability is fragile. It is easy to block it just by the way you see it, use it, by your attitudes, and by the way you think.

43

Here are some suggestions and tips that can help you unlock your idea generation ability. These tips are like brainstorming tools that you can use systematically every time you need new ideas.

The best practical way to have good ideas is just to have many of them first, and then to select the best ones. Generating any idea for brainstorming is focused on just getting the ideas out on paper or onto a screen.

In your brainstorming session you can follow the steps.

First, take a few minutes to think about what it is you would ideally like to accomplish. How clear is the picture you see? Try to refresh and extend your view of the problem. In particular, think of five people you know that come from different backgrounds than yours. Imagine what each of these people, one by one, would see in your problem, and how they would approach it.

Now it is time to start the actual brainstorming exercise. Take a sheet of paper, pen, and your watch. Set a goal to write a certain large number of options for the ideas over 10 or 20 minutes or ideas within a specific short time interval such as a few minutes. A good example is a goal to write 20 ideas within 15 minutes.

What is important in this activity is that what you focus on the quantity of ideas, not quality. When you brainstorm, you just write a list matter whatever comes into your mind, and write fast. You let your imagination flow, and you play. Forget all judging or analyzing, common sense, rules, or practicality.

Depressing, almost unrealistic deadlines play an important role in the brainstorming session. It mobilizes the conscious and unconscious minds. It helps to paralyze your judgment, denounces fear and other mental blocks, freeing your imagination.

Once the time is up, take a few minutes to brainstorm a few more ideas, until you feel that you cannot squeeze anything more out of your mind. Often those last ideas will be the most important ones.

At the end of this exercise you have a long list of ideas, options, and thoughts. You will discard most of them later, at the judgment stage. Yet, the ideas you have tend to be much better than something you would have a logically allowed to follow from what you had in your mind for the brainstorming exercise. The alchemy of results will surprise you, and it is worth every minute you spend on it.

Stress Management

The continuously growing pace of the modern life puts more demand on our stress management skills. You may already be in a situation when you feel pressured to produce more and more every year with less resources and shorter deadlines. Or you may feel overwhelmed by the challenges in maintaining balance between your work and family life while trying to fit in writing into the mix. Whichever sources your stress is coming from, if you just let it build up you will eventually experience some sad consequences. And unless you improve your abilities to deal effectively with stress this may happen much sooner than expected.

How much can poor stress management cost you? Stress has been linked to a majority portion of health problems, from premature aging to heart attacks. Even when stress does not cause the illness directly, it can accelerate development of existing conditions, making you more vulnerable to health problems as well from your home or office environment. And even if you don't count physical health damage and premature death, stress may also diminish a significant portion of your life. Just by keeping you in a state of fatigue, unhappiness, and depression.

Stress management goes hand-in-hand with time management. On the one hand, good time management is a critical element of effective stress management. Time management is probably the number one priority for managing stress. If you get organized, plan ahead, stop questioning, clarify your priorities, and delegate effectively you're much less likely to be overwhelmed by the pre-deadline stress. Even without advanced relaxation techniques. And you're more likely to get ahead in balancing your work and family life and produce some amazing books in the process.

On the other hand, stress management is an essential component of effective time management. Many people cannot completely avoid the sources of their stress, and in overwhelming stress, can block you from thinking and performing well. In such situations, stress management techniques, including relaxation techniques, can be critical for getting unstuck and staying effective. You also need to be well aware of stress symptoms in order to effectively manage your pace in moving towards your goals. If you try to move too fast in the short-term and don't take adequate breaks, your stress may damage your ability and motivation, hurting your longer-term progress.

And it is certainly not a good time management if you become disabled, miserable, or die prematurely from the effects of excessive stress.

Managing your time to succeed in accomplishing your writing goals is what is most important for you. When you don't accomplish what you truly want, you may feel confused, compromise, and frustrated. Many people try to use time management techniques that work for others only to be disappointed. Often this is because they don't also identify the goals most important to them and give you the techniques towards both goals. Effective time management must include techniques for good prioritizing for each individual – not what works for everyone else.

More About Time Management

Before exploring specific time management techniques, consider several common myths for time management, especially since many are undermining your efforts to establish of all your goals:

Myth: my life is completely controlled by external events.
Fact: you can have some control over many aspects of your life, but you and you alone are responsible for initiating the control. Learn to recognize what

you can and cannot control before making your choices. Anticipate the future and clarify the external demands that must be faced. From there, it is easier to determine what can be done, and within what timeframe, despite the demands.

Myth: I should meet everyone's expectations.
Fact: the needs and commands of others may be inappropriate for you and your lifestyle. They may be poorly timed, highly questionable, or simply unattainable. They may be of a different priority than your own. In trying to meet the expectations of others, you may be shortchanging yourself and your needs. First become clear about what your needs are and then consider what others expect of you.

Myth: I should have no limits.
Fact: we all have limits. Failure to acknowledge this may cause you to become perfectionistic in your expectations. Perfectionists are especially prone to procrastination because the perfection they demand is impossible. For example, no one will be perfect each and every way. The long-term consequences of procrastination such as inconveniences, academic or career losses and lingering self-doubts are usually more devastating.

Specific Techniques

While it is important to develop your own style for managing your time and work, consider how the following techniques might help you.

First, stack the cards in your favor. For example:

Use your biological rhythms to your advantage. Identify the times in a day when your energy levels are at their highest and do your most important work at those times.

Optimize your work environment, keep things you need in your work environment. Make sure the physical environment is conducive to concentration, not just comfort. We need to experiment to determine the right work environment. For example, some work best in a quiet setting while others work best with that their music; some work best amidst clutter, or others need a clear desk or table; some with best at a place reserved only for study while others work best at the kitchen table; etc. Find what works best for you!

Second, you need block out distractions during work and writing time. Protect your time by saying no to various interruptions, activities, requests, or persons. Interruptions are a troublesome type: the interruption itself, and the expectation of further interruptions. Both reduce your effectiveness considerably. Some interruptions can be avoided by keeping in mind the following:

- Arrange your work area so that your back is to the traffic flow.
- Close your door; open it for activity only.
- Find or use a special space as such as a library corral or in office an where friends will be unable to find you.
- Unplug your phone, or install an answering machine. Return telephone calls when it is more convenient for you, perhaps when you take a break.

So how can you better balance your work, writing and your life? All these tips will help you find a better balance.

1) Carry out a life review. Take time out to look at where you are currently. Do you want to carry on working the way you are? Do you have enough time to spend with your friends and family? You have enough time for hobbies and leisure time? Why don't you keep a time diary for the week or two to check that you have the time to do everything you want to do as well as reviewing where you could better manage your time.

2) Organize your life. Spending time preparing what you want to do can help you better manage your time both in your job and your life. Every minute you spend planning will help you save time in actually doing the task.

Set aside some time at the beginning and end of every day to organize what you want to achieve and the importance of each task. And at the end of each day review what you have achieved and congratulate yourself.

If the job seems large and unmanageable, first determine what you actually want to achieve. Then, breakdown the goal into smaller chunks into small steps every day until you have achieved it.

3) Learn the art of delegation. Delegation involves you passing responsibly for completing a task or piece of work to another person. It can help them to learn how to complete a task, and enables you to spend time on the other important parts of your work or life. You can eat also use delegation where another person's skills in a particular area are better than yours.

   Delegation includes training someone to do a particular job or getting buy-in from a partner. To effectively delegate in either situation is similar. Decide what you want to delegate. Explain what you want done and the reason is that you need their help. But let go of the past. Give credit for work that has been successfully completed.

4) Review your working arrangements. The average person works 40 hours a week for around 40 years, which equates to 160,000 hours of their life.

   To be truly satisfied in your job, it is important too that the right job is right for you, but additionally that it fits around other arrangements. Many companies offer flexible working, part-time working, job sharing, home-based working, or even career breaks or sabbaticals. This can help to support the other things that are important to you – like writing your book.

   If you feel the review of your working arrangements will help you, arrange a time to talk to your manager and review their options.

5) Look at yourself. Finally, it is easier to achieve work-write-life balance if you are healthy and have time to relax and enjoy your life.

Develop and maintain interests that are not related to work and cultivate relationships with your family and friends. A regular exercise routine, eating healthily and sleeping well can help you to restore your energy and allow you to live a better balance life.

A Shocking Revelation

I'm going to do something that I very seldom do; I'm going to promise you that what you're going to learn in this chapter will, at the very least, double your productivity. Now here's the scary part, the part that almost everyone knows to be true, but that very few are willing to acknowledge: **if you double what most people are getting accomplished each day, you still wind up with a list of things to do most people would be embarrassed to have published**. Let that sink in a little bit. The truth of the matter is that while most of us are incredibly busy each day, most have fallen into the trap that is described as confusing activity with accomplishment.

Some studies have shown that high-level executives, on average, are only actively working on something that can be measured at the end of the day, for 45 minutes. Imagine that, an 8 to 10-hour work day, and less than one hour is actually used towards productively. Are you trying to see why I said that even if we were to double someone's output that it's still not something to be overly excited about? Would they want the whole world knowing how much they were getting done? In the example previously mentioned, we'd still have someone with less than two hours of productive action each day.

But here's the exciting part. I know people are generating very lucrative incomes on 2 to 3 hours of work each day. If you have fallen victim to that "if you want to be successful you have to work 60 hours a week" mindset or relay system, the same people that you know who preach this are the very same people who delusion themselves into thinking that they are working 60 hours a wee. But it put under the microscope, would probably come in at the whopping average of less than one hour of productive time each day. What a waste of life and opportunity to write a book and finish it.

Here's another shocker; some of those people actually have done okay for themselves, so what if they doubled the productivity to two hours a day, and cut out 80% or more of the non-nonproductive activities. Do you think they might enjoy the increase in income, while simultaneously enjoying more free time?

I'm going to reveal perhaps the most powerful technique for converting this into your reality. While there are certainly other techniques that can amplify the impact of the one you're about to learn, this one could truly be thought of as a standalone method.

It's based on the fact that the work we have to do will expand to fill whatever time amount of time we have allowed. I'm sure you can recall the day when you had only had three things to do on your to-do list, but at the end of the day, you were just finishing up that activity. Now, if those three things have been more like 20 things on your to-do list, you would have been able to get the same three activities done in about 1/6 of the of the time; you would've had to if you really wanted to get everything done. Interesting, yes?

When I first started using this method of getting more accomplished, I went back to resolve my to-do list for the previous month. When I took a list that had taken all day to finish and then went back to the rest, assigning an estimated time frame for each separate task, I was shocked to find out that what should've taken me less than 2.5 hours to do what had taken an entire day.

The process is simple - estimate and list everything that you must get done the next day. Make this list even before going to bed; doing so will allow yourself unconscious mind to process the list as you sleep.

After you have made your list, take a look at each item, and estimate how long it should take. For example, if one of your items on your list is to go to the post office to mail some off some letters, you have been there before, so you should have a really good idea how long it will take. Going to the post office for me is 20 minutes round trip, and that's been really generous with the time. Do this for each and every item on your list.

When you're finished, don't be too surprised if you find the 6 to 10 things on your list total less than three hours.

And here's where the rubber meets the road; when you get up the next morning, start with the first thing on your list, do it within the amount of time you assign, and immediately move onto next important task, completing it within the time limit designated as well. Go through the entire list in this manner.

Now, when you find that you have worked through every activity on your list before noon (or anytime during the day), take a few moments to create a new list – list B. This is the list of things you will use the same formula on for the rest of your day. Anything you don't get to, before your workday ends, simply move it to the top of the next day's list.

Here's the short version of this technique:
- Make your to-do list the night before
- Assign an estimated time of completion for each item
- Work through each item in the time allotted
- Immediately move to the next item on the list
- If you finish your work day move on to list B
- Anything from list B that you don't get to goes to the top of the next days list

Remember, you can use this method to either get what needs to be done in a fraction of the time. That way you're leaving more time to use for pleasure or recreational activities, or, if you happen to be passionate about what you do as I am, you can push onto your B list, and move your level of productivity to the next level. The choice is yours; just know that this proven method will work and all you have to do is work it.

Procrastination – the Thief of Time

"I hate doing this task - let me do something else instead which is far less important but more enjoyable and or easier."

Sound familiar? Procrastination is putting a task off to another time where you should be doing right now. It's amazing what we do or will do to avoid doing what we should be doing. It is indeed the biggest success killer!

Procrastination is merely a series of routine bad habits and the lack of discipline. It takes time and determination to change a bad habit.

What causes procrastination? It can be for many different reasons such as: too hard; too compact; not sure where to begin; fear of failure; lack of interest; perfectionism; lack of enjoyment; poor work environment and indecision.

So what should you do about it?
- Break big tasks into small manageable ones
- Reward yourself for completing tasks you do not enjoy. If you don't do it, don't reward yourself!
- Create a deadline: otherwise tasks will usually go on far longer than they need to. Tell others of your deadline.
- Create a distraction free environment
- Complete tasks no matter how small and cross them off of your to-do list. Each little completion will give you momentum!
- Do the toughest, most un-enjoyable tasks first.

Procrastination is the thief of time. It takes away your self-esteem, your momentum, and performance suffers as a result. Many of the above tips on beating procrastination you have probably heard before. It is one thing to know what to do; quite another to do what you know. Follow through some of the suggestions above and you'll see impairments right away both in performance and self-confidence. Good luck!

Why are Some People Much More Productive?

Time is something that we all have the same amount of yet some people seem to get a lot more done in that amount of time than others. Does this amount to some utilizing their time to the fullest extent? The answer is yes - there are several things you can do to increase what gets accomplished in the time you have available.

One misconception is that you will be able to get things done in your free time. I'm partial to the fact that there's no such thing as free time. To get you started, find someone already successful that you look up to and remodel after them. They got what they are for a reason. They set the priorities and organize them to encompass their objectives.

Remember in school when you had to write everything down to remember teachings? When you write down the things that need to be done, then your mind is on a roll with "Now let's get stuff done" and there's no more wasting your time trying to shoot from the hip. The big thing is to get considerably organized.

Many people waste time looking for things to find the particular items they're needing to get their own tasks and writing taken care of. Stacking things for later ends up requiring more time than just getting things filed in place and organized. Use slots to avoid the amount of material stacked on your desk. Successful and productive authors are organized, utilize the skills of others, do not try to take on everything themselves and focus.

Listen and learn about great ways to help keep things in order that you wish to accomplish in any given day. By the end of the day you will have a very good idea of where you will need to begin tomorrow.

Organize Your Reading

Most of us have a fair amount of reading to do at any given time. A lot of authors continue to read snippets now and then of their favorite authors to help generate ideas or just escape a bit.

Mark important paragraphs or sentences should you need to return to them later. It is advisable to keep those resources you need to refer back to available whenever you need them quick and easy access to previously-read material.

When you have errands to run or places to go for your business find a place for errands in similar proximity to avoid going back-and-forth about times. This will increase the usability of your time more effectively. Keep in mind though, that people you visit or see will keep you waiting from time to time. Do your best to utilize the time by having a book or CD handy while you're waiting that encourages work flow. Find ways to avoid letting other people abuse your time. Learning how to say no is very difficult for some people – learn to say thank you but at this time I am unable or I have other another appointment.

Whatever it is needs to keep you from assisting because you know that you're not available. Make sure you're honest, sincere, and firm with your statement and let others know exactly where you stand in that your time is very important to you. At least recognize that it's important to do the task right the first time - how many times have you cut corners to get something done to do it the second time? How much time did you save? Exactly! None, as a matter of fact, it cost you twice as much time in the long run.

Remember - time can be your ally to its fullest if you take only a few steps to get started.

CHAPTER 5: THE WORD OF MOUTH PHENOMENON

The concept of "word of mouth" (or WOM as I call it), the simple act of one person sharing something with others, has been around since the dawn of business. Word of mouth marketing is an attempt to influence and encourage this phenomenon, getting consumers to talk about a brand and recommend it to their friends.

How Worth of Mouth Marketing Works

Studies have found that 92% of consumers trust recommendations from friends over any form of advertising, so it's not surprising that many businesses put great effort into word of mouth marketing. With the advent of social media that allows a single person to potentially share things to with millions, the possible rewards of a word of mouth marketing effort are in many cases astronomical. Having a marketing message "go viral" has, in fact, become the holy grail of advertising.

How Word of Mouth Marketing Works

There are many ways to get consumers talking about a brand. Generally in word of mouth marketing terms, there are direct and indirect approaches.

A direct approach is a "hands-on" attempt to spread the word about a brand, focusing on retaining control of the actual message. An example would be hiring people to join online forums to talk about the brand in a positive light. This can be very effective when successful, especially for a new business that has very little brand recognition to start with, but it also has the chance of backfiring if consumers spot the attempt. Usually it is not taken to kindly, and can actually cause a lot of damage to the brand. Another example would be a referral program that rewards consumers for recommending the brand to their friends.

The other, indirect approach is very common these days. A quick visit to YouTube is all it takes to see this approach in action; fun or controversial videos can be a great vehicle to get consumers talking about a brand. Generally, an indirect approach leaves the brand with very little control over what consumers are actually saying. This can actually be a good thing, as it ensures the discussion is authentic and there's no chance of the campaign backfiring.

What are the advantages of focusing on it?

The main advantage of word of mouth marketing is obvious: a brand that can harness its power successfully will enjoy a steady stream of new customers simply through referrals from their friends. Since these prospects are somewhat pre-qualified (they already trust and like the brand), they'll also be easier to convert into customers in many cases.

Another advantage is that a highly successful viral campaign, designed to increase "buzz", can potentially take a new brand from completely unknown to a worldwide household name in just a few days. That is a rare outcome of course, but even a campaign with much less reach can benefit a brand greatly.

We can expect word of mouth marketing to keep increasing in popularity in the coming years, as it's a way for brands to break through the noise and reach consumers in a non-intrusive way. As consumers get increasingly blind to regular advertising, directing effort towards word of mouth marketing may be the smartest strategy for a brand to focus on.

In the next few articles, I'll be talking about how to incorporate word of mouth marketing into the various marketing strategies such as email, social media and even mobile marketing. In addition, we'll discuss when word of mouth is less useful, what makes an advertising campaign WOM friendly and how to measure the results of your **word of mouth marketing** efforts.

How to Convert Your Existing Customers into Your Biggest Assets

If you were buy a new automobile or mobile phone and a trusted friend mentioned that a particular make you were interested in purchasing had faults but another model was much, much better, if you are like me you would sit up and take notice. This is because consumers trust their friends, family, influencers and authority figures to make recommendations about products and services to them, in addition there are many ways to make recommendations. These could take the form of a testimonial, an affiliate link, a referral, a direct mention from customers, they all work to some degree.

To encourage your customers to provide you with an endless stream of referrals, you can take some steps in advance that sets everything up to turn your best customers into your biggest business assets.

Be the Best You Can Be

The better you do your job, the more pride with which your customers can recommend you to others. If you provide excellent products, services, and customer support your customers will be happy to provide referrals when asked to do so.

Ask Customers to Refer You

Develop a company referral script, that everyone in your company will use, something along the lines of "my business is expanding and I'm looking for customers like you who could benefit from our products / services, who do you know that you could recommend?"... Pause and wait for names and details... "Would you mind if I used your name, when talking to this person or better still could you introduce us? Pause and wait for an answer....

By developing your own referral script and using it whenever you complete a project you will maximize the referrals given to you. It's also a great idea to give customers some literature and information about your offerings so that they can easily share with others.

Create an Active Online Community

Using either a message board, forum, private Facebook group, or even your newsletter it is possible to create a community that can help spread the word about your great services and products.

Build Long Term Relationships

Focus on relationship building over the long term and never risk a relationship to make a quick profit. By doing so you will create true raving fans that are eager to recommend your business. By developing real relationships with people, you're creating fans that are much more likely to tell others about you.

Create a Formal Referral Program

Offer discounts to friends and family recommended by existing customers, along with a coupon of some sort (gift voucher) to the one who gave the referral. With a formal referral program you should let every customer know about it as soon as they become full customers.

Use Social Media

Offer a coupon code for consumers "liking" or "following" your brand on social media, and encourage them to share. Offering sign-up incentives for newsletters and more always helps get the word out about your services.

Market Your Testimonials

When someone gives you a raving testimonial, turn it into a meme, ask for a recording, put it into many formats and then publish it and market it across all channels. Market your testimonials as you could other types of content. Oh, and don't hide your testimonials on a testimonial page, spread them around your website for maximum benefit.

Follow Up

The money is always in the follow up, so always follow up with customers who have provided referrals to you by offering them a discount, a thank you note, and acknowledgement. The more you follow up after a positive referral, the more likely they will be, to continue doing it.

Word of mouth referrals are more than fifty percent more effective than any other forms of marketing. If you want to develop a long term business, the best way to ensure that it really is a long term business is to encourage word of mouth marketing in every way that you possibly can.

Many business owners find after years of being in business that most of their customers come from word of mouth marketing, which lessens the need to expend more time, money and effort on other forms of marketing.

Creating Better & More Effective Word-of-Mouth Marketing

Word-of-mouth marketing is perhaps the oldest form of marketing that exists, not only that it's still one of the most effective forms of marketing. It's just common sense that when someone you know tells you about a great product or great service this word-of-mouth marketing outperforms other forms of advertisements.

Ask for Referrals

If you want your current customers or contacts to give you referrals, it is important that you tell them that is what you want. The more you tell your contacts that you want them to recommend you to others, the more likely they are to do it. Every single business should develop a referral script, which should be used once a project is complete while the customer is still at their highest level of satisfaction. Something like "my business is expanding, who do you know that could use my services and would you mind me using your name?" there are lots of variations you can use, the important thing is to develop your own script and use it.

Provide Sources with Details

A great way to encourage people to give you the ideal type of referrals is to tell your customers and contacts exactly what type of clients you are looking for. That way they can be sure to tell the right people about you and your products and/or services.

Be a Resource Center

The more you can help everyone you come into contact with, even if you cannot service them directly, the more you'll be seen as a resource center. This could be accomplished in person simply by putting different people together, or online via content marketing. People will learn to trust you enough to recommend people who can be your actual clients.

Provide Incentives

I used to be a big fan of providing incentives to your contacts that recommend you to others. Some people have successfully given coupons and discounts to those who have recommended them, with great results. However I am now of the opinion that a more personal reward works best, not all of the time but on occasion and out of the blue.

Push for Those Testimonials

Ask for testimonials from your currently satisfied clients to share on your social media channels, share around your website, and within your sales pages. Once you receive a testimonial there are many ways in which you can use them to get more business, and just like referrals never be afraid to ask for a testimonial.

Build a Community of Customers

One way to really push your word-of-mouth marketing is to build a community of customers who can speak with authority about your products / services and awesome customer services.

Create an Affiliate Program

A really fabulous way to create momentum in your word-of-mouth marketing is to open an affiliate program for customers only. They are the ones who can really speak about your company and the quality of the products and services you offer, they have experienced it after all.

Network Strategically

Many people with whom you have casual contact through networking events can be a wonderful resource for referrals. There are many networking groups that you can join to help you get the word out and I know of lots of businesses that have grown into big businesses doing nothing more than networking.

Word-of-mouth marketing remains one of the best forms of marketing available and one of the least expensive and most fun. All you have to do is live up to your reputation and continue to under promise and over deliver so that your clients are thrilled by your products and services enough to keep the word-of-mouth going.

Measuring the Effects of Word-of-Mouth Marketing

If there is one thing that is always true about word of mouth marketing, it's that it's never easy to accurately track the direct results of it. Short of wiring all your customers with microphones and cameras, there's just no way of knowing exactly what they say to their friends about your product or service. This is precisely why many companies decide to not focus actively on word of mouth promotion – it's just not that easy to prove that they will get a good return on their investment.

There are, however, a couple of methods that can help paint a picture of the effectiveness of a particular campaign (or, how much word of mouth activity there is around a brand in general):

Using social media

With the introduction of social media, it has become much easier to keep tabs on what people are saying about a brand. There are in fact many software tools designed for just this purpose. While looking at people's public conversations about a brand may not give the full picture, it is still one of the best ways to gauge interest and measure the results of a word of mouth marketing campaign.

The main issue with relying on social media statistics is that, according to surveys, only 10% of word of mouth activity takes place online. It's still mostly about offline conversations (75%) and phone calls (15%). Still, it's easy enough to do and usually doesn't cost much so this is often the first step taken.

Using surveys

Another popular method of gauging interest and word of mouth activity around a brand is by using surveys. By simply asking customers what they think of the brand, and whether they have recommended it to their friends, it's possible to get a decent idea about how a campaign is going.

Usually it's a good idea to reward users for answering the survey, as it may otherwise be difficult to motivate them. Unfortunately, that often prohibits them from being completely anonymous, which could lead to slightly skewed results (they may not want to say anything bad about the brand, knowing their answer will be associated with them personally).

Using referral programs

There's no doubt that referral programs can be very powerful motivators to spur word of mouth activity, but another advantage they have is that usually they're easy to track the results from. Since the customer who refers one of his/her friends needs to be rewarded for the referral, it goes without saying that tracking these types of campaigns is easy.

However, this method of measuring results is obviously limited in that it can only show the results from this particular referral program campaign. It is therefore quite useless as a tool for measuring word of mouth activity around a brand as a whole.

These were just a few of the most popular methods available to track results from a word of mouth marketing campaign. Every company or brand will have to come up with their own tailor-made solution that suits their strategy, but using these will certainly be a good start.

Incentivizing People With Referral Rewards

One of the most powerful strategies to spark word of mouth activity is using a referral program. The basic idea is rewarding customers for recommending the brand to their friends and family.

Types of referral programs

There are many different ways to implement a referral program, but the most common (at least online) is giving customers a special link they can share with friends. When one of these friends takes an action, like buying a product, the original customer gets credited a reward for the referral.

Another type is using good old-fashioned coupons. When sending out coupons to existing customers, attaching an additional coupon "for a friend" can be a great way to increase word of mouth activity. Just make sure there's some sort of restriction in place so people can't use both coupons for themselves.

In case it's an offline business, it's usually easy enough to just ask customers who they were referred by (if anyone).

Advantages of referral programs

The first, and most obvious, advantage is that it is virtually guaranteed to increase word of mouth activity as long as the reward is generous enough. People are simply much more likely to recommend a company to their friends (or strangers!) if they, for example, get a cut of however much that person spends with the company.

Another advantage over many other word of mouth marketing strategies is that a referral program has a chance of actually attracting customers who are otherwise loyal to another brand.

There's also the usual snowball effect that is to be expected with word of mouth marketing – one person tells 5 friends, who each tell 5 friends, and so on. The difference is with a referral program these customers are actually more likely to actively seek out others to spread the message to, even people they normally don't associate much with. Increased reach is always welcome!

Any disadvantages?

The main worry with referral programs is that the word of mouth activity will not be "genuine". Take away the referral program and people will talk a lot less about the brand. The question is, does it really matter? That will probably vary from business to business, but the rule of thumb is that if immediate sales are more important than long term brand awareness, then it's probably not an issue.

Another potential problem is if the reward is too high – this may lead to customers actually spreading the word to strangers who simply don't want to hear about it. This is especially true if it's an online product or service, in which case it's very easy for users to "spam" others with their referral link. This needs to be taken into account, and there needs to be a plan of action in place for handling situations like that.

There's no doubt that a referral program can do wonders for sales, providing the reward is generous enough (or, consumers feel strongly enough about the brand, but in that case a referral program is not as important). It doesn't suit every business, but since it's usually easy to implement a basic program and see whether it works or not, there's little reason not to give it a shot!

Brilliant Ideas for Using Cell Phone Technology for Word-of-Mouth Marketing

Since most people are carrying their phones with them at all times, it makes sense to try to utilize this for word of mouth marketing purposes. There are a few ways in which mobile technology can be a great help in increasing word of mouth activity around a business or brand:

Text Messages

Text messaging may be a basic technology, but one that can work very well in word of mouth marketing. Just as with e-mail marketing, the idea here is to sending messages to users that they are likely to forward to their friends. The contents could be anything, and will vary depending on what the business does, but one idea would be coupons and time limited offers.

If the business has a "refer a friend" program, this could also be implemented using text messages. An example would be hosting a form on the website where they can enter the phone number of a friend, then having a customized referral message sent out. In this case it is important to take steps to ensure that the feature cannot be used for spamming – for example it could be limited to 1 message per day and only registered customers would be allowed to use it.

In-app Sharing

Almost everyone has a smartphone these days, and it seems like almost every website and business out there has their own app too. The upsides are many, of course, one of which is the ability to easily and instantly share things from the app with the user's friends. Again, coupons and limited deals are perfect for this. Say you're scrolling through the app for a popular web store, and come across a coupon for a certain product. Right away you think about your friend Mike who said he was in the market for that exact product – a couple of "clicks" later and he has the coupon code in his inbox. It's important to make the sharing procedure as fast and effortless as possible, as users on smartphones generally have very little patience for slow apps.

A photo contest can be a great way to increase word of mouth activity around a brand. The basic idea would be holding a contest where the most fun/creative photo relating to the brand wins a prize. So how does this increase word of mouth activity? Well, one idea would be to require contestants to submit their photo through Twitter, thereby showing it to all of their followers (and potentially many more if it gets re-tweeted). A contest like this can blow up and generate a huge amount of buzz for a brand if well executed.

Just as with all other word of mouth marketing efforts, it's important to experiment and not be afraid of doing something wrong. It pays to be careful with text messaging, however, as there are some laws and regulation in place for those. Otherwise it's all fair game, and the worst that can happen is that the idea fails to gain any traction with users.

Word of Mouth Marketing Utilizing Email

"Word of mouth" is traditionally thought of as something that happens mostly in face-to-face settings. In fact, the statistics support this: a study by Journal of Advertising Research showed that 75% of conversations between consumers about brands take place offline. Also according to them, 15% happens over the phone and "just" 10% takes place online.

That does not, however, mean that it can't be worthwhile to construct word of mouth marketing strategies for online communication methods like e-mail. Even in an online setting, a recommendation from a friend will weigh much heavier than a regular advertising message. It is also to be expected that the percentage will keep increasing in the coming years, as the trend shows that less people talk on the phone and instead move to e-mail, social networks and online chat.

Encouraging eMail Recommendations

In its simplest form, word of mouth marketing with e-mail is just encouraging consumers to share something positive about a brand with their friends. Getting just one in ten customers to recommend the brand to a friend can have a significant impact on growth, so it's definitely worth putting some effort into.

The most common method to encourage recommendations through e-mail is probably having an "e-mail to a friend" link on the website, similar to how many businesses have links to encourage sharing on social media. Unfortunately, these links are rarely used by visitors. It requires quite a bit of effort from the consumer, and there is usually no clear reward for using it.

A potential way around this is rewarding consumers for referring their friends to the website (through e-mail or other methods). This will have a much higher adoption rate, especially if the reward is good, but it comes with a big disadvantage: since the recommendations are technically "bought", consumers will trust them less. If they know their friend gets a reward for inviting them, they're less likely to consider it a genuine recommendation.

Content Creation

Another strategy that can increase word of mouth through e-mail is creating content that consumers find good/funny/interesting enough to forward to their friends. This is definitely not easy, and can take a good amount of experimentation to get right, but in the long run it may be worth it. Consider two online stores: one that sends out a weekly message simply listing new items and what's on sale, and another that puts a ton of personality, fun stories and quirky videos in their newsletter. It isn't much of a stretch to think that the second probably gets forwarded around a lot more.

There's no doubt that e-mail can be a powerful vehicle to increase word of mouth online, but there are also many potential pitfalls. As with all word of mouth marketing efforts, making the recommendations appear genuine will be the hardest challenge. What works best will vary from business to business, and it's important to remember that not all businesses are well suited for e-mail promotion. Usually it works best when there is already an existing e-mail relationship between business and consumer.

Word of Mouth Marketing with Social Media

The advent of social media is probably the most important thing that has happened to word of mouth marketing since the telephone was invented. Never before has it been so easy for people to discuss and recommend products and services to their friends and family. The opposite is also true of course, as a single tweet can have a devastating impact on a business if not properly tended to.

Here are a few tips to help devise a successful social media strategy that encourages word of mouth activity:

Keep the communication going both ways

Too many businesses make the mistake of treating social media as simple one-way communication. Most of the time they're really only using it as a vehicle to broadcast their current offerings, and there's very little personality or "fun" involved. Consumers typically get tired of these types of social media accounts pretty quick, as they feel that they're constantly being marketed to.

A much better way is using social media to actually interact with consumers and encourage discussion. Instead of just pushing out endless offers and updates all day, ask the fans/followers questions! Instead of simply deleting negative posts, respond to them in a light or serious way depending on the situation. As long as other followers see the excellent, disarming responses, a couple of bad posts won't do too much harm. In fact they serve to make the brand even more popular! The trick is just being personable and relatable, even if it's the fan page of a huge multinational corporation.

Make sharing easy

This is more related to the business website. It's essential to make sure sharing is easy and all pages are easily reached through a copy-paste friendly URL (which isn't always the case on JavaScript-heavy websites). Using sharing buttons is a good idea in some cases, but it's important to make sure they're not slowing down the website too much, which happens sometimes.

Don't be afraid of being funny or controversial

It's a fact that most people use social networks to be entertained. They're not there to buy things or view marketing messages. It's therefore important to tailor communications to this. Keeping things lighthearted is usually a good idea, and humor can be an extremely powerful weapon to engage fans.

Most companies are very afraid of controversy, but the fact is that in small doses it can help word of mouth activity greatly. It does require a bit of planning and careful consideration of course. A bit of care needs to be taken so it doesn't backfire or gets blown way out of proportion.

By implementing these simple strategies, consumers will be much more likely to share and talk about the business on social media. It's important to remember that social media is something that requires on-going work. For example, it's not enough to jump on the Twitter account a couple of times per week as people expect much faster response times there. It's usually a good idea to set up e-mail alerts when someone mentions the company or brand, and try to respond to these messages as soon as they arrive.

Business to Business (B2B) Word of Mouth

Traditionally, word of mouth marketing has mostly been focused on business to consumer scenarios. The idea being to create an environment where consumers are encouraged to talk about, and perhaps recommend, a business to their friends and family.

The same idea can, with a few adjustments, be applied in business to business situations. What we're looking for here is creating a "buzz" within an industry or business segment.

The power of the launch

There is little else that can generate so much interest and buzz as an exciting, upcoming launch event. Whether it's for a new product or service, or just something interesting that's happening in the company, with the right approach it's possible to get people talking about it months before the actual event. The trick is coming up with an idea that, even when revealed beforehand in only vague terms, gets people's imagination going. There has to be a feeling that there's something BIG coming.

Some companies in the B2C sector have perfected this approach — a great example is Apple, who has millions of people all over the world eagerly anticipating their launch/reveal events. This same thinking can be applied to B2B, although usually on a smaller scale.

Of course the whole idea falls short if the actual launch is disappointing. Failing to deliver on the promises made will decrease customer confidence in the business, and getting a second shot may not be easy.

Creative advertising

Just as clever or creative advertising can be used in B2C to encourage discussion and increase brand awareness, the same can be done in B2B. The concept is actually similar to using launch events. To stand out and actually spur discussion and word of mouth, the ads could be controversial, funny or simply mysterious.

As usual some experimentation will most likely have to be done to find out what target businesses respond best to.

Referral programs

Here's another technique that is used successfully in B2C, and can be adapted to B2B. Many small business owners have friends who are also self employed, meaning they probably talk business amongst each other. If a business has a lucrative referral program, they may be more likely to recommend it to their friends. Of course, just as with B2C, there is a chance these people may not treat the recommendation as genuine, considering the person gets a reward for each referral.

In many situations there is really little difference between B2C and B2B when it comes to word of mouth marketing. The goal for the business is exactly the same: do something that gets people excited and talking about it. The main difference is probably that a bit more professionalism is expected in B2B situations, and the target audience may be a little harder to reach and impress. Otherwise it's basically the same, and as always some elbow grease and a willingness to experiment is the key to success.

Word of Mouth Advertising is Not Right for Every Occasion

While most brands can benefit greatly from focusing on increasing word of mouth activity, there are a few situations when it just doesn't make much sense to spend lots of time and money on.

When selling commodities

Let's face it: few people are talking to their friends about which brand of toothpaste they use. Unless it's one with very special, niche features, most products are simply too similar and too "boring" to be discussed. No matter how fun or exciting the product is made out to be in commercials, and no matter how popular it is or how well it sells, there's just not going to be much word of mouth activity around it.

Sadly, the one time a brand like this may see a ton of word of mouth activity is when/if they make a mistake or do something bad. Then people will start talking, but it will probably not results in more products sold.

When selling mostly through direct marketing

A great example here is products that are sold through infomercials. These companies aren't at all focused on word of mouth marketing – they want sales and they want them now. In fact, many of them would probably prefer it if people didn't discuss their products, especially if it's a low-quality product being sold at a high price.

Of course, word of mouth may still prove valuable to them if they sell a useful, high-quality product, but it's never going to be something they focus actively on increasing. One thing that's interesting about infomercial products though, is that sometimes the actual product (or presentation) will be so strange/funny/unique that word of mouth activity will increase just from that. Those are quite rare, however.

When selling high-end (or very expensive) products

While a few well-off people might buy a private jet based on word of mouth, it's generally not something that the companies that make them focus on stimulating. They're not going to introduce a referral program to get people talking about them on Facebook, because that simply wouldn't make sense (and that's probably not even where most of their customers are).

When selling products or services that are in extremely high demand

Think "rental apartments in a crowded city". People would do almost anything to get a nice, affordable apartment in major cities, and the companies that rent them out are probably not too worried about increasing word of mouth activity. In fact, they rarely have to care about marketing at all – customers will just magically appear whenever they need them!

These are just a few examples of situations where word of mouth isn't something that should be prioritized. It is important to note, however, that just about every business in the world could benefit from increased word of mouth activity, even if they're not actively focusing on it. Sometimes it's just a direct result from selling a great product/service. And, as always, there are exceptions in every industry, and every business is different. There might one day be a company that sells toothpaste based only on word of mouth marketing – you never know!

Friendly Advertising – Making it Memorable

Launching an advertising campaign that spurs word of mouth activity is no easy feat. Most of the TV ads seen running day after day are created with that exact goal in mind, but how many of those are actually memorable or worth talking about? Not many…

There are a few basic ingredients that can be used to create an advertising campaign that gets people talking. Not all of them have to be used in the same campaign, of course. Most of the time just focusing on one of them will be enough. Here they are:

Controversial ads

Nothing sparks discussion as much as a little bit of controversy. It's important, however, to remember that there are two distinct types of controversy: good and bad. The line between isn't always obvious unfortunately, which is why it's important to think twice and be extra careful when choosing this strategy.

Humoristic ads

This is a staple of TV and radio ads. Probably more than half of those are trying to create interest and spark word of mouth activity by being humorous. The problem is, humor is very difficult to get right when it's combined with a commercial sales message. Most of the time it simply falls flat. When implemented correctly, however, this type of ad can have consumers remembering it for the rest of their lives. Maybe it's not surprising that so many brands try this type of ad?

Quirky ads

Here's one that can be almost as effective as humoristic ads, but also one that is harder to define. A quirky ad is one where a viewer (or listener) asks themselves afterwards what it really was they saw (or heard). Get it right and they might even turn the volume up the next time it appears to try to make sense of it! Just as with controversial ads, there's a slight risk of going overboard with this, although a quirky ad is usually much "safer" (but arguably not as potent).

Annoying ads

Everyone has at least one ad they remember that they always HATED when it came on the TV or radio. However, chances are they still remember the company that ran the ad. Furthermore, they probably talked about it with their friends, creating brand awareness and fulfilling the purpose of the ad even if they hated it! It's a bit sneaky, but there's no doubt that it can be effective. As usual, it's important not to go overboard and create something that actually repulses people. A slight annoyance is more than enough!

These were just a few examples of ads that create a lasting impression on consumers, and (hopefully) get them talking about the brand. If increased word of mouth activity is the goal, these types of ads are infinitely more effective than regular "Buy 2 get 3" types of ads. Since advertising is everywhere in our society, standing out and taking a unique position is becoming increasingly important. Companies that fail to realize this and adapt their advertising campaigns to modern standards that encourage word of mouth marketing risk falling behind.

The Encouragement Factor in Word of Mouth Marketing

While word of mouth marketing is undoubtedly powerful, choosing the right strategies for your business may pose a challenge. This article aims to show you a few of the best methods you could use to increase word of mouth activity from your customers.

Before taking steps to focus on word of mouth marketing, you need to make sure there is a solid foundation in place. Even the most amazing marketing campaign will struggle to make an impact if consumers simply don't like or trust your brand. That's why every word of mouth marketing campaign should begin with a thorough look at your current offerings and customers. Is there anything you could do better? Anything you could do to separate yourself from your competitors and make your business the one people recommend to their friends?

You also need to realize that word of mouth marketing isn't an exact science. It can be very difficult to predict consumer behavior. All you can do is make sure the aforementioned foundation is in place, and then implement the following strategies to get some word of mouth going:

Adjust your advertising

If you want people talking about your brand, your advertising needs to reflect it. This is why you see so many funny commercials on TV. Even though they do nothing to directly increase sales, they get people talking and create positive associations around the brand. Depending on your business, however, you may want to keep some of your traditional sales-focused advertising too, and try to find a balance between both types.

Use events to get people talking

Let's say you're an online store and you're about to add a whole new series of products. You basically have two options: you can just go ahead and add them, then send out a newsletter telling your customers about it. This will do nothing for word of mouth activity. Your other option is turning this into an event. You set a launch date, and do your best to get people hyped up for the launch. If you do this correctly, people will start talking and word will spread about your launch. Of course, for this to work there needs to be something really unique or interesting about the new products.

Consider adding a referral scheme

"Refer a friend" schemes can be very successful in increasing word of mouth activity, but they come with the built-in downside of being less trusted by consumers simply based on the fact that an incentive is offered. Still, they can be an excellent source for a steady stream of customers and sales.

If people aren't talking, start the conversion yourself

If you're trying to get some word of mouth activity going online, you may have to get the discussion going yourself. It is, however, extremely important that you don't go around posting fake "reviews" or things like that, as people will most likely see right through it. Instead, one idea might be finding communities related to your business and using your expertise to help out. Soon enough people will start recognizing you, and your business will become better known and talked about in the process.

Don't be afraid to experiment!

Every business is different, and you never know what will work best for you unless you're willing to try (and sometimes fail and try again and again). Unless you're being actively dishonest with customers, the worst that can happen is that an initiative fails to gain any traction, in which case it's simply back to the drawing board!

CHAPTER 6: HOW TO ADD YOUR SKILLS & TALENTS TO YOUR MILLIONAIRE FORMULA BY EDUCATING OTHERS

You can put your knowledge to work and teach others your craft. Are you looking to make money from home, but have no idea what to do? Then consider selling your expertise online; musicians, cooks, life coaches, teachers, and crafters can all sell their knowhow. Today there's a multitude of online platforms that allow you to set up shop and instruct via phone, email, and/or video chat. Most platforms allow you to set up shop for free, accept payments, and even market yourself.

Many professionals, regardless of their education and profession focus so much on 1:1 sessions with their clients, not realizing that the real money is when you can get multiple people in the same room, charging them all the same rate, and making $3,600 for the hour instead of $60. Teaching creates amazing income opportunities, and I advise you to get started on developing a class for your community and clients to take immediately.

Classes can be as easy as "The Best of _____", where you can teach people who want the best of whatever subject you're an expert on. Or, a "How to _____" and utilize your education there.

If you'd like to make money online selling your expertise, here are 11 online platforms to check out.

1. BrainMass

BrainMass is an online academic academy where experts can make money by assisting university, college, and high school students though an online library, one-on-one help, or via their e-book library. Experts must be working on, or have obtained a graduate-level degree from an accredited university. To get started, register online, watch a training video, take a quiz, then send in your credentials and proof of education. Once you're approved, you'll be able to generate content for BrainMass. The academic expert pay rate works on a sliding scale. Payments are paid on the 15th day of the following month via PayPal or check.

2. Clarity

Clarity is an online marketplace where people can sell small business advice to entrepreneurs. Simply create a profile through LinkedIn, set your rates, link up your PayPal account, and wait for calls to come in. Topics you can speak on are Business, Tech, Sales and Marketing, Funding, Product Design, Skills and Management, and Industries. Clarity hosts over 30,000+ verified experts, including Mark Cuban, Eric Ries, and Cameron Herold. Clarity takes take 15% of the fee collected from the call and you get the rest. Payments are made via PayPal every 15 days.

3. Createpool

Createpool is an online marketplace for information selling in the following areas (pools): Programming, Academics, Auto Repair, and Legal Advice. To become an expert, create an account, search online for questions, give advice, then make money. Createpool deducts a 20% service fee from each transaction and payments are made via check or PayPal.

4. Ether

Ether is a company that lets you sell advice and content by phone, email, or through your website. Sign up for a free account, then set up your Ether Phone Number where calls will be forwarded to you. Set your rate and hours, and answer questions, Ether takes a 15% fee of what you make. Payments are made via check and direct deposit. Some examples are a therapist, doctor, nurse, tax expert, teacher offering their expertise to customers.

5. Expertory

Expertory is an online platform where experts can sell their knowledge through live online video chats. Often referred to as "The eBay of Learning", Expertory gives professionals a platform to market, schedule, accept payments, and instruct individuals all in one place. Totally free to join, you decide when and where to teach, and how much to charge. Expertory doesn't take a cut until you've been paid and fees will vary depending on where the referral comes from. Expertory has been featured on The Washington Post, USA Today, and The Charlotte Observer.

6. Helpouts by Google

Helpouts by Google is an online platform where you can sell your expertise in a variety of subjects and fields. Sign up by creating a Google Plus account, choose a category, fill out your profile and price your expertise — then start selling. Google will take a 20% fee and the rest is yours. Payments are made via Google Wallet.

7. LivePerson

LivePerson is a unique service that connects individuals who have questions to people who are qualified to answer them. Here's how it works, LivePerson has all the backend tools in place, so once you've completed your application and set your fees, you'll be connected to people who need your expertise. Answers can be delivered via live chat, email, or phone. Once the action is completed LivePerson takes a percentage of the fee you charged then pays you the rest via check on a monthly basis. LivePerson has been featured on The Huffington Post and USA Today.

8. Maven

Maven is a micro-consulting platform that allows you to profit from your knowledge and connections. To get started, sign up for an account, select an hourly consulting rate, and answer some questions, which are sent to you through the Maven match-up feature. Payments are made via PayPal, check, and direct deposit. Maven charges a $4 – $25 fee per month based on usage. Maven is a member of the Better Business Bureau and has been featured on Forbes, the Wall Street Journal, and The New York Times.

9. Odijoo

Odijoo is an online campus that allows users to sell their knowledge in a couple of ways. The first is to create an online course and sell it through Odijoo, they deduct 10% from the purchase price whenever someone purchases your course, then you keep the rest. The second way you can generate revenue is by creating an Odijoo campus classroom, where you have your own private online space for training people. Campus seats are sold in blocks, with each seat representing one user taking one course. Seats start at $7 per seat along with a $2,000 annual setup fee. It's free to create an account and payments are made via PayPal.

10. Popexpert

Popexpert is an online video portal where you can sell you knowledge on Meditation, Marketing, Music, Relationship, Career Mentoring, Language, Nutrition, Productivity, and Style. Set up your profile, set your rates for a 50 minute video session, let others know your availability, then instruct your lessons via video. Popexpert's fee is 3% when you have a session with a client and when they refer a new client to you, their fee is 20%. Popexpert pays will transfer money into your bank account 21 business days after your video session has ended. Popexpert has been featured on USA Today, Mashable, and the Daily Muse.

11. Udemy

Udemy is an online teaching platform that allows individuals to teach on a variety of subjects (business, design, art, education, music, etc.) Instructors create their content, publish it on the site, and then promote it. As an instructor you'll set your rates and promote your classes for which you'll receive 100% of the revenue. If a class is promoted through Udemy and a sale is made, they keep 50% of the revenue. Using Udemy is free, except for a small processing fee for accepting payments. According to their site, most instructors make an average of $7,000 annually. Udemy has been featured on Mashable, the Wall Street Journal, and The New York Times.

CHAPTER 7: IT STARTS WITH SERVICES & PRODUCTS

If you were to win a large amount of money and then decided to invest a good proportion of it, would you expect your financial advisor to invest it in just one stock? Just like investing, earning business income should not be done from a single source. When you invest, you choose a wide variety of different stocks (businesses) in which to invest in, in order to leverage any loses to a minimum. This is the approach you should aim for with your business income, if you can diversify the places from where you can earn, and the types of products and services from which you can earn you'll accomplish the same thing.

It doesn't matter what kind of business you have, or what your target niche is, you can multiply your earnings by creating multiple streams of business income.

First we create a service or product and then we figure out different ways to make money from it, as a business owner you understand this. You could for instance off a wholesale price for your product to distributors, or perhaps a bulk order discount on services, you can sell your products yourself from your website (I hope we designed it) at full price or if it's a physical product maybe also in a store.

You could also look at affiliate marketing and it's always best to start with existing customers, affiliates are businesses who will promote the products and services you offer for you, in exchange for a commission on sales.

Most experienced business owners could write a book, and open up a coaching or consulting business. You could even teach a class about your specialist topic. These are all different income streams surrounding the same product or service.

You want to have a good mix of active income and so called passive or residual income. Active income are activities you perform directly to earn revenue – such as providing a service like coaching, writing, administrative work and so forth. Passive income is when you do work once, and are paid for it indefinitely. This would be something like writing an eBook or information product, or selling memberships to a club or members website.

I've actually taken this a step further and combined both an active and residual income together in that I rent to clients websites (residual income as I design it once at the start) and then I provide ongoing monthly services (active income) this, in my opinion is the best form of income.

The wonderful thing about earning money from a multitude of sources is that if there is a downturn you're in a much better position than most. As most business owners could in theory write a book, let's use that as an example.

Your Book: How to ABC

Sources of income for your Book How to ABC:

Direct book sales

Product recommendations via blog and book

Consulting/coaching with people who want to do ABC

Speaking at events about ABC

Teaching courses about ABC

Selling other people's related products

Advertising relevant ads on your blog about XYZ

Writing for magazines about XYZ

These are all legitimate ways to make money just by writing one book, I am sure you can think of others. The book could have been born out of another money making activity such as being a contractor, virtual assistant, writer, graphic designer, internet marketer, or something else entirely like a health and nutrition expert. Whatever your niche you can make money doing the things listed above, creating multiple streams of income that far exceed the potential income from just one activity, this is the secret to true success.

The idea of multiple steams of income works for bricks and mortar businesses too. If you sell a widget retail, you can now offer it wholesale, and attract affiliates to sell for a commission, thereby creating three streams of income from one product. You could expand that further by writing a book, recommending other products, consulting with others and so forth.

It's not hard to create multiple sources of business income once you start considering all the ways you can earn from one product or service, the real secret however is in actually doing this.

Services

Freelancing

Join a freelancing site and offer assistance as time permits. You can bid for jobs and have your employees do them. Or, you can find an eBook that you've already written on the subject the client is looking for and offer to sell the rights to it.

Coaching

You can do online coaching live or pre-recorded. If you want to maximize your time, opt for pre-recorded coaching sessions that are based off of a book that you've already written. Sell your coaching sessions off of your website.

Training

Offer training through your website by explaining a difficult concept or how to do something you're an expert in. You can also do training as an eCourse or in a live class setting, and charge people a substantial fee to learn from you. I've known some classes to bring in as much as $50,000 a pop and fairly large conference rooms were used.

Consulting

You can offer consulting on a 1:1 basis or pre-recorded. You can provide consulting products and sell them off of your website. You can write a book and label yourself as a consultant if you've provided assistance to others for a fee.

Speaking

Speaking engagements bring in a lot of money. My recommendation is to never do them for free. If people want to learn from you and your experience/education, let them pay for it. Speaking requires a lot of preparation and time.

Events

Events are great ways to draw attention to your brand. Attend tradeshows, fairs and such to stay in the public eye. Hand out promotional gear or branded merchandise to gain followers and trusted clients.

Design

Have you designed something? Let others pay for the rights to use those designs. Photographs are an excellent example, but maps, graphics, infographics, measurements, specs, etc. are all valid design elements that can have a price tag put on them.

Donations

Donations received from your website can also be a form of revenue. I've known a major dad blogger to accept donations for his site to keep running. You can have people pay your hosting fees for you with a simple link asking for money.

Products

Virtual Products

Courses — sell courses and teach from your blog! This is the easiest way to repurpose your content and make money. Online courses are high in demand and people want to learn how to do something that only you know how to do (very well). Put it online and sell it!

eBooks — these are the goldmine offering of any website. You can use them to get email subscribers (to build your audience and selling capability) or you can use them to draw in income. Make sure they are well-written and edited for mistakes and grammar.

Software/Plugins — hire a freelancer from another country that works for cheap to build you an app that compliments the work you do and the experience you have.

Audio — develop an audio series that people can listen to at work or in their car or even at home about things you are an expert in. Sell them from your website and upload the CD to any print-on-demand CD manufacturer or service provider. Throw them on Amazon.com to sell and you have another income stream!

Video — create videos on how to do something you love to do that help people at home or at work. Sell your videos online through your site and make it part of a membership package or a paid site access-only section of your website.

Webinars — schedule webinars that are either live or pre-recorded. Teach your viewers about a subject you're an expert in and how they can improve their own situation. Charge a fee for admittance.

Reports — Write a report that has beneficial information in it for colleagues in your field to use to help them with their jobs or provide info that people online are looking for. Hint — check forums and unhappy customers with a brand and provide a solution!

Physical Products

Books – Everyone is capable of writing a book, but whether it's a good book or not is the ultimate question. Spend time and expense at writing the book and use an editor. Sell it on Amazon.com and Barnes & Noble.

Merchandise – Sell products you obtain at wholesale at retail price.

DVDs – Sell training DVDs or DVD-Roms with software you've had engineered or content on them. Put them on your website or sell them on Amazon.com or eBay.

CDs – Sell CDs that contain music that supports your brand, have music mastered that is original to your brand, offer an audio CD of you speaking on a topic, or have a CD offering digital products on it.

Branded Retail – Your brand on t-shirts, mugs and mouse pads is great advertising. Find a product your clients tend to need or enjoy and find a manufacturer printing company that will supply them to you at a wholesale price.

Get the Idea?

See – everything related to your field of expertise can be branded and spun into a paid product or branded merchandise item. Don't make the mistake that millions of entrepreneurs make and not see these projects through. Use the skills you learned in Chapter 4 about time management and start these projects right away. You'll start earning income immediately.

CHAPTER 8: EFFICIENCY & PRODUCTIVITY

How Recycling is a Lot Like Content Repurposing

Recycling is perceived by many as being an environmentally friendly act. There is however another element to recycling that is often overlooked, recycling is an efficient and cost effective way of reusing a resource.

Just look at paper and aluminum, both of these items are interwoven into the functioning of a modern lifestyle. However, aluminum and paper are both expensive to extract from the natural environment. Despite this extraction cost, the price of both substances needs to be kept to a minimum. If the cost goes up, the price of things containing aluminum and paper rises to a point where they are no longer affordable. When this happens, that functioning, modern lifestyle begins to grind to a halt. In short, people need aluminum and paper but don't want to, (can't) afford the extraction cost it takes to obtain them.

The answer to this problem is recycling. When used aluminum and paper are recycled, the great cost of extraction is balanced out by the relatively cheap cost of recycling. This results in more aluminum and paper being available at a price acceptable to the average consumer. So, at this point, you may be asking yourself "What does any of this have to do with content repurposing?" The answer is simple, everything.

Content repurposing is a lot like recycling. In fact, content repurposing is exactly like recycling when it comes to efficiency and cost effectiveness. Let's face it, creating original, high quality content is a difficult and expensive process. It's difficult because information presented in a logical, clever and engaging format requires large amounts of research and thought. It's expensive because all that research and thought takes time and, as the old saying goes, time is money.

The cost of content creation, in this sense, is exactly like the extraction cost for aluminum and paper. The time and effort of creating content is so high that it stops many people from content marketing altogether.

Content repurposing, again like the aluminum and paper example, balances out and reduces the high cost of content creation. This means that content once again becomes "affordable" for the average business person engaging in content marketing.

Now, by affordable we don't mean purchase price, what we mean is that content repurposing allows the average person to be able to drip out repurposed content to their target audience simply by changing the way the original content looked or read. So, the next time you reach for a paper product or a cool drink in an aluminum can, remember content repurposing and how it can make your content creation needs easier, quicker and an awful less stressful.

Using Your Resources – Human & Digital – to the Max

As a busy business owner it can seem almost impossible at times to get everything you have to do, done. Do you look around at others and wonder how they get so much done and make it all look so easy? There are some tried and tested methods for getting more done each day that you may not have considered as an business owner.

Delegate

No matter how large or small your office, even an office of one you can still delegate both work and the tasks you might have to do at home. Hire a virtual assistant to help you with all those mundane repetitive tasks that aren't your main money making ones and especially the ones you don't like doing. It might be checking your emails and dealing with customer service, carrying out blog post research, social media activities, doing business research, preparing monthly reports and it might also be housework. It's up to you what you delegate, the secret however is to give up some of that control and free up your time to do the things you do best.

Use Your Calendar

Today we have so many useful ways to use a calendar. Using an online calendar that lets you create separate calendars for each portion of your life yet integrate them into one big life calendar (such as Google Calendar), can be a very good way to keep track of your schedule. You should also aim to schedule not only work tasks, but personal time too, this is especially important as you need time for yourself if you are to achieve more.

By scheduling work in time increments that you think you need to get a particular task done, you'll be able to fill your calendar more productively. For instance, if it takes you 15 minutes to check email in the morning, schedule only 15 minutes for checking email. By micromanaging your calendar, you'll end up with more time to do everything that matters to you.

Set Milestones and Deadlines

When you do services for others it's simple to create milestones and deadlines based on your clients' needs. But, it can seem a little harder when you're creating milestones and deadlines for yourself. Even so, it's an important component to being more productive as it's stop you exploring other avenues as they arise and makes you focus on the task at hand. Be realistic when determining how long any one project should take you. Then, work your way back on the calendar to today giving yourself enough time each day to work towards meeting your milestones.

A Little Self-Discipline Goes Very Far

Periodically during the day, double check yourself to ensure that you are doing tasks that are in your calendar. If you're not, stop what you're doing, look at your full calendar and start working on the things on it for today. Do not allow yourself to do anything else until you've done the things on your calendar for today.

Reward Yourself

Just as tasks should be listed in your calendar, so should rewards throughout the day. Put into your calendar "when I finish xyz I can spend 15 minutes reading this blog and learning something new." Set a timer so that you don't lose track of time. By keeping track of your time this way, after about a month it will all become second nature to be very productive and not let yourself get side tracked.

Create Checklists

Do you do something on a regular basis over and over again? Do you have a new client checklist? Do you have various task checklists to ensure you don't miss a step? Many different professionals have checklists that help them stay on track for any one task. They use it to ensure that nothing was forgotten. Don't assume you'll remember; use a checklist every single time for best results and I've personally learnt this the hard way, losing hours of time simply because I forgot one step in a long process, checklists stop this and save you time they are also extremely useful when delegating to people, as they can follow your checklist.

Finally, always stay mindful of the consequences of being disorganized and unproductive. As an entrepreneur, everything rides on your ability to be able to plan, organize and implement all the tasks and projects you need to do on any given day, week, month, quarter and year. As you create processes and implement them, you'll be amazed at how productive you'll become.

Productivity is the Key to Becoming a Millionaire

Lack of productivity is something many of us suffer with. When you work at the office, it's very easy to get distracted by everything going on around you. And when you work from home, productivity can unfortunately be even more of an issue.

Here are a few tips designed to help anyone who is struggling with their productivity levels.

#1 – Stay focused. This is easier said than done, but one sure way to boost your productivity is by staying focused on one task at a time. Studies have shown that those of us who "multitask" actually get less done. Having your email program open along with several other windows on your computer is very distracting and will take away from your ability to focus on the task at hand.

Try to do one thing at a time. If you're checking your email, stay focused on that until you finish. If you're doing your accounts, give yourself a set amount of time to only work on that task before moving on to something else. And if you find that you struggle to stay focused on one task for very long, then simply give yourself a set amount of time to work on that one task. It's better to give yourself fifteen set minutes to check email than to look up an hour later and realize you haven't gotten very much done.

Staying focused on one task at a time really does make all the difference to your productivity levels.

#2 – Write a list. Lists can be a very positive tool when used correctly. The trick is to write a realistic list of the things you would like to accomplish during each day. If your list is unrealistic and includes too many tasks, you'll only feel disappointed when inevitably you haven't checked off all the tasks at the end of the day.

So stick to a realistic, succinct list. You can always add more to it if you're very productive on a particular day. Once you have your list then take it one task at a time. Stay focused on each individual task until you finish, then check it off your list.

#3 – Take a break. Now this may not seem very productive at first glance, but did you know that people who take regular short breaks tend to be more productive than their sedentary counterparts?

A quick five to ten minute break every hour or two will help you recharge your batteries and get your energy levels flowing again. During the time do anything that makes you feel better, but ideally you'll want to completely step away from your desk and do a few stretching exercises. A few deep breathing exercises wouldn't hurt either.

If you have time and feel up to it, a quick two to three minute stroll will help you feel energized and ready to focus on work once again. And don't forget to drink some water. It's a well-known fact that dehydration can lead to sluggishness and simply feeling "not quite right." Avoid this by regularly drinking water throughout the day.

Staying focused and productive can be simply a matter of breaking down large tasks into manageable ones. It's easier to do this when you set realistic goals for yourself and stay on track by writing a to-do list that, again, is quite realistic.

Taking Breaks

Are you working and working but just can't seem to focus and get stuff done? You might be considering changing careers or even seeing a doctor, but the solution may be much more simple than that – just take a break. Taking short ten minute breaks throughout the day can help you refocus and reenergize so you're more productive once you get back to work.

Scientists and psychologists have actually done many studies that show how effective breaks can be. In fact, many large businesses have now started adopting break times into the course of the regular day. Employees are actually paid to sit at their desk and read, research topics they enjoy on the Internet, and do other things that interest them. It's been shown that allowing these breaks actually increases productivity and employee satisfaction enough to compensate for the lost time plus some.

To get the most good out of your breaks, try making your activities something that will help increase production when you return to work, rather than something that simply distracts you. Some great options include aerobic activity or relaxation exercises. They'll clear your mind, while producing chemicals in your body that will boost concentration when you get back to work.

If physical exercise isn't your thing, or you just don't have the chance to do it at work, there are other things you can do to relax and clear your mind so you can get back to work. Meditation or other breathing exercises only take a few minutes, but can help you feel better mentally and physically. Not only does it help you focus, it can also lower your blood pressure and help reduce the physical signs of stress.

The biggest danger in taking breaks is not getting back to work when the break is done. A lot of people will try to skip breaks because they're afraid they won't get back to work and the work won't get done. But when you skip breaks, you can significantly decrease productivity and actually end up getting less work done. The key is setting a time limit to your breaks and sticking to them. If you have trouble, try setting a timer when you take a break, or having someone back you up by making sure you get back to work.

If you've been pushing too hard and have reached burnout, a ten minute break just isn't going to be enough. If you are finding yourself feeling sick, tired, and only ever in a negative mood, especially about work, you are probably burnt out by work. In this case, you not only need to incorporate short breaks into your day, you also need to alter your how and when you work and may even need an extended vacation.

Breaks are an easy and effective way to increase your results and become more successful with very little effort.

Get Automated with Marketing

Marketing automation is essential for online marketers. It's not just a nice thing that adds to your productivity; it's absolutely necessary and there's one simple reason for that – It takes over routine menial tasks for you so that you can focus your time and energy on more important things.

Saving Time for "Thinking Work"

As an online marketer, what should you be spending your time doing on a day-to-day business? Your true role as a marketer is to study your market, and plan and execute marketing strategies. In other words, it's "thinking" work.

However, when you're bogged down with simple routine tasks that anyone (or any machine) could do for you, you're losing that precious thinking and organizing time. The hours you could be devoting to really careful consideration of your brand image or mind mapping your overall marketing strategy are wasted away on busy work.

Get Routine Tasks off Your Desk

In addition to planning and organizing, another important part of marketing is building relationships. You need to be actively engaged and interacting with the members of your target market, whether on social media sites like Facebook or Twitter, or through face-to-face offline events or online webinars.

Relationship building, like planning and organizing, takes time. Also, relationship building tasks cannot be done by a software program, an outsourced worker across the planet, or a nifty gadget. This is work that you and only you can do.

If you can successfully automate routine tasks and get them off your to-do list, you can spend more time interacting with members of your target market, and the benefits to this are priceless.

We're all being pushed to do more and more, productivity is one of the key elements many businesses are looking at improving, with everyone driving themselves mad trying to do more things at one than is humanly possible. You might call this multitasking but the truth is, it's a myth that multitasking is effective. If anything, multitasking is costing you big time. By some studies, multitasking is showing a decrease in productivity by 50% or more.

Multitasking Makes You Lose IQ Points

Whenever you try to do more than one thing at a time it actually makes you perform at a capacity similar to being drunk. Whatever you are doing, business, sport or parenting you get about as much from it, as you put into it. So, if you focus and give 100 percent, you'll get 100 percent back. Just like those old samurai films which mention how they used to give 100 percent to everything that did, this is how you need to be.

Multitasking Restricts your Creativity

When you can let go of the noise around you, you can also become much more creative. It's very hard to get into a flow if your phone is ringing, you're constantly checking and answering emails, or the beeps and the dings of social media are interrupting your train of thought. You not only need time to truly focus on a project, but you also need time to focus elsewhere between projects to kind of clear your brain of the noise a bit, before moving on to the next thing you have to do.

Multitasking Is Dangerous

Not only is multitasking dangerous for your health in that it can make you stressed and even ill, but it's also dangerous to your safety. If you are driving and talking on the phone, you are putting yourself in grave danger that's why it's illegal. You would not get behind a wheel drunk, so don't get behind it and do anything but drive. Likewise when it comes to doing anything, focus on the task at hand and you'll be less stressed, which will translate into being healthier.

Your Brain Isn't Designed to Work that Way

No matter how you want it to work, no one's brain can really focus on more than one thing at a time. Yes, of course you can talk and walk at the same time, but texting and talking is not something you should do. Writing a letter, spending time with your kids, focusing on data entry, making sales calls… all should be done one thing at a time. If you learn to make your to-do list with this in mind, you'll get more done faster and your work quality will go through the roof.

You Need 15 Minutes to Adjust to a New Task

A Microsoft study showed that when you're interrupted by something like an email message, a beep from a phone, or by someone physically interrupting you, it can take 15 minutes to get back on task, meaning to get back into the flow where you're doing the task at the highest level that you can do it. It's important to keep this in mind as you plan your day if you want to perform at your highest capability.

Don't fall for the popular misconception that multitasking is an ability that you should strive for. It's just not a good idea for anyone to multitask, it's bad for your brain, it's bad for your health, the work your produce isn't as good as it could be, and it just isn't really possible to do.

Technology is changing constantly, in fact if you follow the technology news sources you will find that it's constantly evolving and being improved upon. This means that there are a great many tools out there that can help reduce your workload and increase productivity. Using the right digital tools can help you automate lots of tasks and simplify your job in numerous ways. Let's jump right in and look at how you can put technology to work and make the time you spend at work a little easier.

One of the best ways to reduce your workload and to make your life a little easier is to look at using an online project management tool, these are really a must have, when it comes to keeping up with who is responsible for what task, tracking those tasks, storing files and procedures and keeping everything organized. There is absolutely no question about it, if you have multiple projects in the works you need to be using this type of tool in your business.

When your workload is starting to become overwhelming and you know there isn't enough time in a day to get it all done, it's time to seek some help by outsourcing some of your work. There are some great websites that will allow you to easily outsource, and to start with I would advise anyone to outsource to locally based people, because outsourcing overseas is often a challenge in itself.

Other tools you may want to consider are the online productivity tools. Some examples of these are Mozy, Dropbox, Google Calendar, Google Docs, Asana, Hootsuite and Zoho. You definitely want to ensure you have a backup storage method, a way to stay organized and keep yourself and your team focussed and on track. There are a multitude of online productivity tools that are used for many different reasons, you just need to find the right tools for you and your business and determine what works best for you.

If you find yourself constantly posting on your blog, Twitter and Facebook, you will want to use an automation tool of some sort to make this easier. The tools can save you a great deal of time in that you won't have to constantly copy/paste between the platforms. There are many different automation tools you can use based on your requirements that will make this a lot, lot easier, I know I use some of them myself with Hootsuite being a favourite time saver.

If required you can even schedule your blog posts and social media posts to appear at certain times of the day or night. This can save you a huge amount of time, because you can pre-select these postings and you will be seem to be active on your blog and social media while you are in reality doing something else.

You'll also likely need to utilize a file sharing service such as Dropbox, Amazon and Evernote. These sites allow you to share documents and files with everyone you are working with. Having this facility at your disposal will help you keep your team on track when it comes to completing assigned tasks and managing projects.

As you can see, there are many different technology tools that can make your job easier, lessen your stress and automate your business tasks. This will save you lots of time and help keep you and your team on the right track and I can assure you that the tools above are just the tip of the iceberg with new tools coming out daily there is bound to be one, just right for you, ask on your favourite social media channel what others you know are using.

If you work as a freelancer or as part of a small team, improving productivity can mean the difference between earning a good living, taking on additional clients or not. But if you can establish a good workflow for the type of work you perform you will be able to take on more clients, work smarter, faster and make more money.

For a Better Workflow Develop Package Rates

It never ceases to amaze me the number of people that sell themselves based on a certain number of hours, for example I'll build you a website and it should take me thirty six hours and my hourly rate is $100. The client accepts the hourly rate and the contractor then monitors the time taken on the project and bills accordingly. Instead of doing this, look at offering packages based on your experience, then you can avoid the tedious task of having to track your time. Time tracking for multiple clients, with lots of interruptions can be a massive headache that you don't want, if you can avoid it.

Value Based Selling

I know this article is about developing a good workflow however one of the biggest advantages of moving from a time based billing system to a package one, is that you are beginning to sell based on value and not time. This means that as you become more experienced, the value you offer your clients can far exceed that offered by your competitors and you can charge accordingly, something you would find hard to do on an hourly billing cycle.

Create Checklists for Each Project

When you do the same types of project over and over again, creating a checklist to help guide you and more importantly others who work with you through each project will help keep you keep on task and keep your standards high. Remember, pilots use checklists every single time they fly, to avoid forgetting something, you should too, as it's the smart thing to do.

Deliverables First

Before crafting your workflow, focus on your deliverables firs,t and then work your way backwards to today to figure out what needs to be done first. Then start with first things first, using your checklist to ensure you don't forget something adding what you need to do to the calendar.

Draw Your Workflow

Seeing a workflow visually can help you identify areas that you left out or forgot. You can actually use the checklist for a generic project to create a workflow. For instance the workflow for publishing an eBook might look like this:

Research the niche > Develop a topic > Craft a title > Outline the book > Write the front matter > Write the end matter > Design a book cover > And so forth.

When you draw it instead of write it, you can more easily see the things that can be done simultaneously and what has to be done in order.

Use a Project Management System

Using a project management system like Basecamp.com, or Teamwork.com is a good way to get yourself and your clients organized from day one, I personally use asana.com a lot as it is really good at allowing me to create workflows and checklists. Each system already has some ways to organize the work so that you don't have to actually create everything from scratch.

Use Other People's Workflows

You don't have to start from scratch, do a quick Google search for "workflows" and then fill in the topic such as self-publishing, writing an eBook or writing and publishing, and you can find workflows that are already written. While you cannot sell those, you can use them and modify the ideas for your own use privately.

Try Out Your Workflow

Before considering a workflow set in stone, try it out from step one with a real project of your own to ensure that you didn't leave something out. This is your chance to improve it before asking someone else to try it.

Ask Others to Try Out Your Workflows

Send the workflow to someone else that you know who also works on the same type of projects that you do, whether it's someone on your team or a colleague, asking them for feedback, advice and tips on improving your workflow.

Refine and Improve

Nothing is ever perfect and this means your workflow is actually never set in stone. As technology improves, and clients' needs change, your workflows will evolve. That's what's great about drawing them out and creating them in the first place. Your workflows, over time, can only get better.

Workflow design is essential to your success as a contractor who takes on the projects of multiple clients. Ensure that you develop your workflows based on the services that you offer so that your project management practically runs itself over time and so that you always know where you are and what you are supposed to be doing.

Many business owners understand the importance of social media marketing, however they don't understand the work involved, before embarking on any social media marketing campaign it helps to have a strong team behind you. You need competent staff to help with all aspects of your social media marketing campaigns, from creating the content you'll share, to physically posting the content to meet your scheduled requirements, as well as developing marketing and engagement campaign ideas. But, if you don't really understand the technology, how can you be sure you're hiring the right team members?

The hardest part of the hiring process is actually prospecting for potential team members, you can of course do this in a number of ways. You can create a job description for each position you're seeking to fill, that outlines the main duties, responsibilities of each as well as a list of daily tasks the team members will be responsible for, then simply allow people to apply for the position.

Alternatively, you can conduct a search for the right candidates by asking your colleagues, or by wading through profiles online to find someone you want to be part of your team. And don't forget the tried and tested method of poaching someone from a rival company that is already doing a good job. It's up to you how to proceed but once you have a few prospects and candidates, why not put them through a few paces to see how well they really know and understand social media, and how communicative they'll be with you if they think you're wrong about something.

After all, you want a vibrant team that isn't self-contained. You want them to speak out and tell you something is crazy, won't work, can be made better, and so forth. Unless of course you really do want little robots who just do what they're told and if you do, you won't have any real success online. In that case, move along and keep on doing what you're doing. But, if you really want to staff your social media team well, keep reading.

Don't Put Your Eggs All in One Basket

Don't seek a wonder woman or superman to perform all the tasks that need to be done. Seek instead several people to handle various aspects of your social media marketing campaign even if this means hiring them on a part-time basis.

If you are particular active, you may want a separate person for each social media account. This accomplishes two goals. One, you aren't tied down if you really don't work well with your choice. It's just one social media account; you can handle that until you find someone else. Secondly, you want someone who is an expert in that particular social media. There are so many things that can be done on each type of social media, that no one person can know them all.

Let Them Prove Their Worth

Ask them to use the social media that you are hiring them to handle to show you why you should hire them. If they are to be your Twitter expert, then they need to show you how great they are, and what an expert they are at utilizing Twitter to get attention.

The same applies with any other social media someone is claiming expertise on. They can show you Twitter growth reports based on a case study as an example of what they've done in the past that shows their worth, or they can do a publicity campaign to get people to vote for them for the job.

Choose a Great Company

If you don't want to go through all that, or manage a team yourself, you can choose a social media marketing company that already has a team in place. Find two or three companies that you like, and openly let them know who you're considering for the position and what your expectations are.

Ask them to explain to you how they're the best company for the work in comparison to the other company. What do they offer that is so different? Let them point out how they can differentiate themselves from the competition, and pick from there.

One further thing, please make sure you speak to me, especially if you have a reasonable budget and want to do great things, I especially looking for companies wanting to capitalize on content marketing utilizing Twitter (mainly), Facebook, LinkedIn and Google+ ... have a look at this typical Twitter report and then see what our competitors generate for you.

CHAPTER 9: HELPING OTHERS & MAKING MONEY AT THE SAME TIME

5 Reasons Your Business Should Support A Charity

Many small businesses take the opportunity to get involved in their local community and give back. Nonprofits and charities are constantly looking for funding to help accomplish their goals, and giving can be really beneficial for your business. Besides, your company's success doesn't just include the one ingredient of your hard work. It also includes all the loyal customers who could be a part of local nonprofits and charities.

But picking a charity is not as easy as it seems. Set aside time to research an organization that fits your company culture and values. Then, think about what charities your customers support. Review additional factors such as the frequency of donation periods.

No matter what you choose, here are a few ways giving back can help your small business.

1. Tax Deductions

Your business can claim your volunteer hours and contributions on your income taxes. By itemizing your deductions, you can write off any time your business spent volunteering and you can add monetary value to any donations given as well and claim them, too. Make sure you are working with a nonprofit organization that is approved by the IRS. The only way to get the most out of these deductions is to have a record with the charity's name and the donation amount or amount of time you worked.

The types of donations that are tax deductible include volunteered services, sponsorships of charities or events, donations of inventory or services, and cash donations. In general, you can get deductions of up to 50 percent on your adjusted gross income when you follow the tax code closely and incorporate charitable giving into your business model.

Companies like LUSH Cosmetics have always made giving back to their community a core part of their mission by selling products where a certain percent of the sale goes to one of over 400 grassroots charities they support. It not only gets the company involved with giving back to their community on a large scale but they also offer the opportunity to their consumers to help.

2. Employee Benefits

Employee perks have escalated to new levels in the last few years, with start-ups leading the pack with yoga days and catered food. Increasingly, people can choose to be picky about their workplace, given their qualified skillset and experience levels.

In a 2007 study by Deloitte on volunteering, 62 percent of 18-26 year olds questioned "would prefer to work for a company that offers volunteer opportunities [to their employees]." What this means for your business is that you have a better likelihood of attracting the type of candidates you want working for you if you offer these types of experiences.

Getting your company involved with your community is great way to boost morale and keep your employees happy. Giving your employees time to participate in events during work hours is fun for the whole business. Not only does it give everyone the opportunity to interact outside of the office space but it also allows them to feel like they are giving back to the community that has supported your business.

3.Free Publicity

Sponsoring a program and volunteering your business's time are a great ways to not only raise awareness about a specific cause but also promote your business in partnership with an organization or event. You can get the word out about the event by posting on your social media platforms and your website.

Kabbage does one volunteer project each quarter and posts news, pictures, and information about the Camp Twin Lakes and other projects on the Kabbage Kares section the website. Taking pictures of your charitable endeavors is a great way to generate press for your business and the cause you are volunteering for. Chances are the nonprofit you are working with will also promote your business on their website and event signs by posting your logo. Lending your brand to a specific cause is a great way to convey your company culture and values to your community.

4. Gain Customer Support

Giving back to your community will help you gain massive traction with your consumers. A 2010 study done by Cone Communications revealed that 85 percent of consumers have a better outlook on businesses that give back to a charity they care about. This means it would be valuable for you to do some market research to identify the most backed causes in your area.

Hook & Ladder Brewing Company out of Silver Spring, Maryland, took this concept and really made it work for their business. They started a program called "A Penny in Every Pint," which donates a portion of beer sales to local firefighting communities, focusing on burn treatment and awareness.

Participating in programs like these shows your customers that you truly do care about your community. Using some portion of your profit for good is a great way to rally the support of your consumer base.

5. Giving Back is Good For You

The best benefit of having your business support a nonprofit charity is the feeling you should get from giving back to others. You have the power as a community to stand up against poverty, human rights violations, and more. Organizations like GLIDE, Make-A-Wish, and Junior Achievement make it possible for your business to give back to your community.

So meet with your employees and find out their interest. Join your community and fight a cause that means something to them. Choosing the right charity that will truly give you the full benefits of working with a nonprofit, so get involved, get your employees and customers involved, and really try to make a difference in your community.

Speaking of Community, What's Your Story?

Telling your unique story starts with these questions:

When, Why and How Did You Start?

The best way to show authenticity is to be able to tell your audience when, why and how you started doing what you do. If you can tell your story so that your audience relates to it, depending on your skill it's also possible to draw them in and get them to root for your success. By doing so you will be able to pull on their emotional heartstrings as you'll be perceived as a close friend, almost part of the family so to say.

How Do You Want Customers to View You?

As you write your story, it's important to convey ideas, values, mission and aims in a no-nonsense way that isn't perceived as fake and contrived. While your story might not engage everyone, that doesn't matter and isn't important as they are not your audience. Your audience consists of the people who can relate to your story, who share your values and want to be part of your story.

Where Do You See Your Business in the Future?

This is where you get to dream as big as you want, let your audience know where you see your business in the future. Whilst doing so you can also refine customer expectations towards what you offer rather than what the competition offers. For example, if you donate a percentage of profit to a particular charity, people should know about it.

Answering these questions is important, it defines who you are. You are going to be able to share this with your audience, via every communication you have with them, be it your blog, social media or through the types of products you offer. With the answers to these questions you can start to form your story and weave it throughout everything you do.

- **Share through Story Telling** – This might be hard to do at first, but persist until you are comfortable using an honest, no holds barred communication style to tell your story, your customers story, and the story of your products and services is a great start. Use interviews, case studies and in-depth blog posts to accomplish this.

- **Share through Doing Good** – Something else you might want to share and blog about is your involvement within your local community, how you give something back that is noticeable and if you aren't doing this then you should be. You don't want to do this just to get noticed as that will come across and work against you. But you do want to pick something that helps people to understand who you are as a business owner and what your business stands for.

- **Share through Experiences** – If you've been around the block you and your audiences will almost certainly share many common experiences that should be discussed. The more ways you can relate to them, the more they will relate to you and the more ways they'll see your products and services as being unique and different.

- **Share with the Truth** – Given how almost everything is spun nowadays you might be tempted to exaggerate, hype and blow smoke, these tricks aren't needed especially as people are smart to such things. All your audience wants is the black and white, warts and all truth. If it takes twenty hours a week to do what you do, and you're teaching them, tell the truth. If you've had to stay up all night to work around your wedding anniversary, say so and if you turn fifty just like I did the other week and you decide to take a day off, share that too.

- **Share Everywhere** – Many business try to share their story in a fashion on their about us pages. You should however tell your story everywhere, use infographics, memes, blog posts, guest blog posts, articles, testimonials and every possible way you can think of to spread your story. More importantly be your story by your actions.

Your story is unique to you, to your brand and is weaved throughout everything you do. It showcases your values, ethics, your past, present and future, and it makes you stand out from the rest in a compelling, relevant and useful manner. By sharing your story you will increase your ROI exponentially as people will connect with you like never before.

CHAPTER 10: WRITING THE EBOOKS & CHANNELING AN INCOME STREAM THROUGH CREATIVITY & KNOWLEDGE

The first time I ventured into the scary realm of ebook writing, I had to Google how to do it.

Seriously. But with the growing demand for businesses to publish ebooks to expand their reach, I figured that do or die I was going to get it right. Since then, I've learned a lot more about what works and what doesn't, and I've written multiple ebooks for my clients. Here's my recipe for producing a successful ebook, in 7 fundamental steps.

Step #1: Define the Target Market

This is a crucial first step in anything you write, but even more so for an ebook that takes longer to write (and costs a lot more money) than the average blog post. The more narrowly you target your niche, the more likely you are to get results. Start with a broad definition of whom you're writing for, then break it down into segments and create personas.

Let's assume you're writing an ebook to attract subscriptions to a tour operator's mailing list:

- Does the company target travel agents or travelers?

- Are the products (tours) offered high end and expensive, or backpacking and budget?

- What are the demographics of the customers who typically take up the tours available?

When you've listed and grouped your targets into various categories, decide which group you're *specifically* targeting with the ebook and create a persona with a name, a job, a life and needs, wants and desires.

Step #2: Identify the Call to Action (CTA)

Ok, now that you know whom you're writing for, you need to determine what you're trying to tell/sell them. Usually the client determines this, but if you're a marketing writer for a company you might be the one in the hot seat. Remember, ebook writing (and any other form of content) doesn't work well unless there's a clear CTA that tells the reader exactly what you want him/her to do, and what they can expect to receive in exchange. In an ebook, you'll likely have several different versions of the same CTA appearing in various locations to reinforce the message, so make sure that you know what it is and that you write content that supports it.

Step #3: Select the Tone, Size and Format

This might sound obvious, but you'd be surprised how often I ask an ebook writing client this question and they don't know the answer! You can't just start writing and hope you reach the end somewhere. I've found that good questions to ask the client are:

- What is the primary purpose of producing the ebook, e.g.: create awareness/generate leads/brand building?
- What are the main points you want covered? Even if a client doesn't have a clue how to go about ebook writing, chances are good s/he knows roughly what they want in it, so don't accept only a working title.
- How in-depth do you want the information to be, e.g.: brief overview/general explanation/detailed instructions?
- What's the main message you want the reader to take away from the book?

The answers to these will give you an idea of how much information you need to provide on the topic and how to break the information up. Your target market definition should help you to pinpoint the tone and format, too.

Step #4: Create an Outline

No, I don't just mean a list of the chapters or sections. I mean what goes into each section, too. You have a specific message to deliver and by now you know what your CTA/s are going to be, so one way to structure the ebook for maximum benefit would be to create sections that each support a different question or objection the prospective customer might have.

Map out each section in terms of the format, the information that's going into it and the projected number of words. This will help you to identify whether the "size" is realistic, too.

Step #5: Write the Intro and Conclusion

Yes, I know we all learned in school to write the essay first and the intro last, but that doesn't necessarily apply to ebook writing. You can "tweak" them later, but by writing the beginning and ending first (based on the outline, naturally) you create a framework for yourself to operate in. You're less likely to find yourself going off-track in the midst of a chapter, because you can keep referring back to your intro and ending for information. Say what you're going to say, say it and then say what you've said.

Step #6: Let it Rest

I never, ever turn in an ebook writing assignment right after I finish it. Not even if I've proofread it *twice.* The reason is because fresh eyes see things that tired ones don't, so let your work—and your eyes—take a break of at least a few hours to a day before you finalize it.

Step #7: Check and Finalize

Once your rest period is over, review the content and weigh up carefully whether your writing delivers on the promise in the introduction all the way through. If not, you can either modify the intro or the body, but there's nothing worse than an ebook that starts off saying one thing and ends up saying something else. Read it aloud—that will help you to pick up typos as well as awkward phrasing and ensure that when you submit it to your client, it's the very best work you can produce.

CHAPTER 11: ACCEPTING OPPORTUNITIES & DOMINATING THE MARKET INSTEAD OF SURVIVING SLOW MONTHS – CHEAP PPC MARKETING

Every business no matter what their size has slow times of the year, generally when their clients are on vacation or when tax bills hit for example. This means that you need to be able to fill this void, while they are gone so that you still earn money even when your customers are on vacation. There are ways to fill the time and avoid issues of this nature entirely.

Ask for Advance Notice On Long Term Contracts

Put into your long term contracts a request for a minimum of a 30-day notice if your client plans to take a vacation without continuing to pay you or provide work for you to do. Explain that you will fill the time with short-term work and projects. Most people are happy to provide notice because they understand that this is so that you can fill the income gap.

Have a Short-Term Sale

As soon as you have a client tell you they're going to take a vacation, arrange to have a short-term sale to fill the time. Make the sale limited, focused, and based on the time your client will be gone so that you don't end up overworked instead of just filling the space. You can create sale packages that you only send out to your contacts each time a client goes on vacation.

Build Your Passive / Residual Income

All service providers should consider building up their passive income so that when one client takes a vacation or some time off, it doesn't matter. Start a side blog with affiliate sales, create a paid eCourse or membership site, or write a book. There are many options to help you create side work that creates recurring income.

This is a favorite of mine, consider structuring your business so that instead of collecting a large upfront fee you collect a monthly fee, this gives real residual income and I do this with website and website marketing services and this has ensured my business is prosperous all year round. You could look for similar types of opportunities in your business.

Avoid Anchor Clients

An Anchor client is any one client who pays you 40 percent or more of your monthly income. Anchor clients are tempting, but they are a bad idea because you are going to be too reliant on the income from that one client. If none of your clients comprises more than 10 to 15 percent of your income, you can easily cut back on expenses and use the free time to work on your own projects without worrying about money.

Work Only on Retainer

Another way to avoid issues with clients going on vacation is to require a contract that is based on a monthly retainer fee being paid by subscription on an automatic basis. The fee can be made so that it is a minimum amount with a minimum set of hours you make available to the client that does not roll over. Without the paying of the fee, your client can't request work from you.

By using these tips, or a combination of these tips, you can avoid losing money when your client goes on vacation. Create solid contracts, be ready to have a sale, build up your passive income, avoid anchor clients and if you are in high demand, consider working only on a paid in advance retainer basis.

Keywords for Your Pay-Per-Click Advertising

Whenever you undertake to run a PPC campaign, selecting the right keywords is a crucial part of having a successful campaign. Over the years I have watched lots of businesses waste thousands of dollars using inappropriate keywords often turn what would otherwise be a successful campaign into one that loses money. It's therefore important to understand what type of keywords you need to bid on and why.

Don't Use Broad Match Keywords

Broad match keywords are set by default, and most people make the mistake of bidding on keywords using them. A broad match keyword means you want to bid on a keyword like "content marketing", if someone searches for "content" it will assume "marketing" or if someone types in "marketing" it will assume "content." It basically shows your PPC advertisement to as broad a range of phrases that have some relation to your chosen keyword phrase. This isn't the way you want your searches to work, especially if you have a limited budget.

Use Exact Match Type Keywords

An exact match keyword is as the name suggests an exact match to the phrase you entered, using our example "content marketing" a user would have to type "content marketing" for our PPC campaign to serve an advertisement. Exact match keywords are what I would suggest most people new to PPC use, as I consider them to be the best because it makes you research the best keywords to you, as well as your audience so that you can select the best keywords that will work.

Choose Fewer Keywords per Campaign

Instead of bidding on every keyword or keyword phrase that you can think if, choose one, two or three phrases per campaign. By doing so, you are using one of the best methods to ensure that the right people find your products or services at the right time. It works on the principle that you do a lot of research to determine what these keywords are, and because your campaign is so focused and you're using your budget on just these highly targeted phrases you will do lots better.

Find the Right Keywords

Use a keyword tool such as Google Keyword Planner or Keyword Tool, which is a good alternative to Google Keyword Planner. Once you've chosen your niche, you can start finding the best keywords to market your products. You want to find keywords that are low competition and in high demand. This means people are searching for them, and there isn't a lot of supply which obviously increases the cost per click. These keywords will be your most lucrative yet less expensive, you just have to spend the time finding them.

External Links:

Google Keyword Planner – https://adwords.google.com/KeywordPlanner

Keyword Tool – http://keywordtool.io/

Test Your Keywords

Try your keywords to see if they work, run a test campaign to see if your targeted audience clicks the ads, joins your email list or buys your product. If all those things don't happen, then you should choose a different keyword. You want keywords to attract the right people at the right time and not competitors or people looking for a job vacancy.

Keywords are an essential element in your marketing efforts, and especially pay-per-click marketing. However, it's also important you, remember that you are creating content and products for people. The people who are your target audience have desires, needs, hopes and dreams and problems that you need to solve. Never forget that.

PPC Methods that Work

I know of lots of business owners that have tried and given up on pay per click (PPC) advertising mainly because they have tried to make it work and failed. I also know of many businesses using the services of an outside agency which is great if you find a good one that really understand their stuff but it's a waste of money if you find a poor one.

Pay per click campaigns are however higher effective if they are well planned and executed and almost anyone can successfully implement them, and achieve success if they have realistic goals. Let's have a look at a few PPC tactics that work well to improve your business when PPC is implemented.

Remarketing

Remarketing is not just for big businesses, small businesses can also remarket just as effectively. It works by signing up with an agency such as Remarketing.com, Google or even Facebook. They will provide you with the technology, which is generally a piece of code you insert into your website, this puts a cookie on the computer of the person that has visited your website, and who has not converted into a customer. Then, when the visitors goes to other websites within Google, Facebook or any of the other remarketing websites, they will see mention of your website. Consider this, someone comes to your website, they visit the contact us page (the page with the remarketing code) and then leave, only to visit Facebook later in the day. Whilst using Facebook they see your remarketing advertisement and think to themselves, that reminds me, I was going to contact them today. They click your advertisement and make contact. That is the promise remarketing offers, it targets people already interested in your company with advertising.

Build Your List

Instead of using PPC to try and sell actual products which at times can be hard, instead consider using PPC to build your list. You might offer something like an eBook, discount coupon or something else of perceived value in exchange for an email address. By building your list, you are putting yourself in a position where you can marketing all of your products and services to them over time, instead of trying to sell just one, straight away.

Local Targeting

It doesn't matter if you have a national or international business, local targeting is a good thing to do. Write content that is focused on a particular location that has a high amount of your target audience within it.

Segmentation

When you plan your PPC campaign you want to set realistic goals, for each goal you will them want to segment your target audience down as small as you can and then create at least one advertisement for each. You can also use the tools available to target only certain people with the ads that you create, but you need to know who precisely these are.

Make Awesome Landing Pages

When you plan your PPC campaign you should create special landing and sales pages for each advertisement. This helps ensure that you target the people that you want to target, not just with the ad that they click, but on the page they land. Sending them to the front page of your website might help you generate visitors but chances are it isn't helping you hit those goals.

Test Everything

It's important to test everything in all forms of marketing however with PPC advertising it's imperative. Even if you've loads of experience with PPC advertising you still need to test to see what works better. The easiest way to do this, is to try two different PPC ads targeted at the same audience with slight differences, one might have a different headline, or a different call to action. By doing this you can see which one works better, until you are happy with the results. You might also try the same ads on a different audience… the important take away here is to always test and measure.

Audience First

It's all too easy to focus on the technology, the content and the keywords, but never forget that first and foremost you're marketing to people, and people have emotions, thoughts, feelings and the ability to differentiate between a good and bad deal.

Numbers Count.

You need to monitor your numbers, even if you believe your campaign is working your numbers will tell you. At various stages during your PPC campaign, compare the results with your goals. If they are not lining up then you need to make adjustments to your campaign to try and put it back on track. Numbers tell you exactly what is what, never ever run a campaign without checking them as they might also indicate small tweaks that if made can make an under performing ad suddenly start to outperform others.

Every small business should nowadays be able to run a successful PPC campaign especially with all of the tools and help available on Google, as well as the social media giant Facebook. But, as with most things, before you start work out some realistic goals you think you can achieve and ensure you can perform from a business point of view if these are achieved. There is nothing worse from a marketing perspective to have a successful campaign running only to have the website fail, or to run out of stock of that product and not be able to fulfill orders. Set realistic goals, measure, change, be prepared, get ready, and go.

CHAPTER 12: SOCIAL MEDIA

Starting Out in Social Media

Starting out in social media marketing can be both daunting and exciting. On the one hand you have a fresh start for your business online; a blank page to be filled, and on the other hand, blank pages can cause writer's block and cause you indecision.

It really important to realize that first impressions count just as much online as they do in what we have come to know as the offline world.

Neither do you have all the time in the world to try out every social media platform for size. Your social media marketing campaigns need to produce measurable results.

Getting started isn't something you should worry unduly about. There are six criteria you can use to help form a coherent marketing strategy.

Decide what networks to join

The big players in the social arena constantly shuffle for first place and they nearly always seem to hit the news with their latest leap in popularity, but the same six players are key in terms of volume of users – Facebook, Google+, Twitter, Instagram, LinkedIn and Pinterest.

Understanding the demographics of each platform's users and where they intersect with your target audience will decide for you whether you should enter a specific social media platform or not.

Decide who's in charge of posting updates

Chances are, you're going to need a virtual assistant to look after your social media. The internet doesn't sleep, and if your market is global the chances are you will have to state your business hours publicly and hire someone to engage with your fans or customers from 9-5 each day.

This is one time when giving the job to your newest intern is not a good idea. Your social media manager should have a firm grip on best practices, customer service, and be both polite and patient as they are the best asset you have online.

Research and plan what to post

It's strange, but sometimes what we actually think our customers want from us and what they actually want from us can be miles apart. Do your homework, figure out what kinds of posts go down the best with your target audience and give them what they want, remember its always about your audience and never about you.

Always monitor your analytics to both help create more of the content that gets the most engagement and to look out for trends your business should follow.

Make a decision on advertising: paid or free?

If you're a new business, or have been badly affected by the downturn in global economy, you may not want to invest in advertising. But understanding how it works can offer some very cheap marketing opportunities, as social media advertising is the most cost-effective there is at the moment, in my opinion however you need to understand how to make it work to generate that return on investment.

Understand how to deal with negativity

Unfortunately, being on the other side of an anonymous void, armed with a keyboard can make some people feel they can do and say what they want with some degree of anonymity.

This is actually a myth thanks to the many different social search tools and aggregators online. Don't feed the trolls that come to cause trouble. Remain calm and make use of the immediacy of social media to offer customer service in a timely and friendly manner. You may never appease the originator of any negative comments, but the world that watches may be impressed enough by your attitude and response that they will choose to do business with you in the future.

Plan on how to benefit from the growth of your customer base

There's little point in growing a large list of fans or followers on any social media platform, unless you leverage it by engaging your followers and encouraging them to share your content. Create some fun around your brand; offer quizzes, photo ops, competitions, fill-in-the-blank slogans. Anything that surprises your fans with an engaging activity. Even companies that sell washing powder have done this by sharing specific tips on how to best use the washing powder for certain types of stains.

Whichever social media platform you decide to use, don't be swayed by size alone you'll be spending a lot of time there, so also follow your passion. Different social media platforms have differences in gender and age group that more than make up for overall numbers, so make sure you also do your homework first and create a realistic customer profile that fits with the social media platform you choose.

Think of social media like you would any other business event where you meet other professionals in your line of work or complementary business. How you behave at a networking event is pretty much how you should on social media: a mix of friendly chat, brainstorming and business. It's too easy when you sit at a keyboard to forget that the person reading your posts, tweets or updates are people too. It's wise to remember that words spoken (in this case typed) in anger or frustration are publicly visible on the social network in question.

Never allow yourself show negativity when using social media for business.

By following this simple rule, you will achieve a much higher level of networking than if you were to gripe and moan about every little niggle, setback or perceived slant you encounter online. Remember too, that words can be misconstrued and that's why someone with great wisdom invented those little emojis that make updates so much fun.

The precautionary rules don't stop at being positive. Avoid gossip like the plague. No one wants to do business with someone they can't trust, so if you earn a reputation as a gossip the chances are you'll never find worthwhile business partners.

Don't rant about competitors in a public space, and don't do the opposite either. No one will respect a self-appointed fanboy (or fangirl) who just hangs out at their profile page like it's the lap of God.

So, you're upbeat, positive and ready to mingle – now you just need to approach a few others at the party. But who should you connect with?

Luckily, online it's a lot easier to figure out who has influence than it is in real life. Rolexes can be faked, tuxedos can be hired for one night only, but true online statistics don't lie.

Before we find the top people in our industry, it's important to understand what keywords we will use to search for them. This applies context to our search. There's little point in connecting with indoor heating specialists if we are an ice cream company. Context is everything.

Let's take a look at six sites which allow you measure your potential joint venture partners' sphere of influence so that you can figure out whether you are a good match for business.

We want to determine who the influencers are in our industry for two reasons: to get them to follow us back, and to connect with their followers.

Here are six (of many) ways we can find influencers:

- Twitter.com – search for your keywords and use the Riffle Chrome extension to view the number of followers each prospect has

- Buzzsumo.com – search for your keyword and check the 'influencers' tab for the people whose posts have been shared the most for your keyword

- Klout.com – Explore your topic and the top influencers' Twitter accounts will appear down the side of the page to your right. You can even follow them without leaving Klout.

- Wefollow.com – Simply search your interest and you will find the most prominent people on Twitter.

- Followerwonk.com – Another Twitter search engine, this one shows those who have tweeted your keyword, how many tweets they have tweeted, how many people they follow, number of followers they have and a score of their social authority marked out of 100.

- Google Plus – Circlecount.com is an awesome tool. You'll need to start your research elsewhere, but when you want to check up on whether a person is active on Google+ you can find some great info here such as how many users are in the circles they share to.

Regardless of niche or platform, you can instantly spot the people who are serious because they always have a complete profile.

Gathering your list of influencers is the first step, next comes outreach. We need to build a real relationship with those people. Notice I said "real relationship." This is what social media marketing is about: building relationships, not yelling "buy my stuff, buy my stuff" or trying to trick people into something they wouldn't normally want to be a part of. Remember the analogy at the start – where we are using social media in the same way as we would press the flesh at a real world networking event or party?

Starting with sites like Twitter is fine, but short updates and tweets aren't big relationship builders. They do allow people get an idea of who you are and what you are about so that they can choose to deepen the relationship on a site like Facebook or Google+.

Here's how to catch their attention:

Add value to the relationship. Don't try to create a friendship just to get something out of it. Do it to help other people. Doing so will demonstrate that you know your stuff and are willing to help others out without being one of those people who will only ever do something if someone pays them.

Be creative. If an influencer doesn't understand something that you do, find imaginative ways to help them understand. You need to stand out in someone's mind to move from a name on the screen to a real person at the other end of an email or phone line.

Don't make it all about business. Try to find common ground with your prospect. Most of us take kindly to people who share our passions and if that means you both share a love of 1950s tin car toys, it engenders an "us against the world" instant camaraderie.

Respect other people's time. Just because someone has had a degree of success in their field doesn't mean they owe you a free consultation.

Enthusiasm is contagious. If you can be positive about your message and give more than you take, just as in real life, you will attract others to you on social media.

Using Pinterest to Help Your SEO

The ultimate aim of engaging in any social media interaction including Pinterest is to drive people to your website. The secret to Pinterest is to include enough engaging information to get your target audience to not only re-pin your pin, but also to follow you so that they can re-pin and share more of your pinboards, enabling them to click through to your website for more information.

There are a few tricks I can share with you for accomplishing traffic generation using Pinterest.

Create Themed Pinterest Boards

Your website blog should be split into keyword categories; you should create a new pinboard for each category on your blog. Additionally, create some pinboards that are lifestyle oriented for your target audience that don't necessarily go along with your blog, but match the interests of your target audience. For example, if you have a bookkeeping business and your target customers are beauty shops, you might, in addition to the typical tips and information about bookkeeping, include a board for new hairstyles or products related to beauty shops.

Include a Quote from a Blog Article

Within the description, include a quote or summary of the blog post that you will be linking your readers to. This will engage them and perhaps pique their interest enough to get them to click through. Be sure that your blog posts or articles and description resonate with your audience and match the particular theme of the pinboard you're attaching it to.

Choose a Relevant Image

Create or purchase an image that will go with the topic, is interesting to look at and brings meaning to the words, in the article or blog post, your image is the first thing people see so try and engage your audience. The image is also a good place to put a quote, a logo and URL watermark, and other information relevant to the blog post that you'll be linking to. Images are of extreme importance on Pinterest. There are several software programs you can use to help you create images fast, like Canva.com and Pixlr.com.

Link Directly to Your Blog Article

Don't just link the pin to your homepage, that's a rookie mistake, instead link directly to the exact page that you want your readers to click through and read. It can be a blog post, a landing page, or some other content and even a product if you wish. It's up to you. The point is, you want the link to go to your site, not someone else's. Even if you are promoting someone else's products and services, lead them to your site, then to the product or service.

Finally, don't shy away from long images like infographics, or from using video. Pinners love infographics and they love watching video. Anything that is highly visual and pretty to look at will entice them to go further to see more by clicking through to your information.

Like most online marketing, it's important to understand how to maximize search engine optimization so that you can get the most out of your time using **Pinterest for marketing purposes**. You can pin all day long, but if you're not optimizing for keywords and using an effective keywords strategy, you might be wasting your time and will never get any sort of meaningful results.

Pinterest SEO Tricks

Before you make your first Pinboard, think about what your goals are for Pinterest and how you want to appear to the world. You've likely already researched keywords and hopefully have hundreds to choose from, at least initially try and select long tail keyword phrases, these are slightly longer phrases that aren't searched for quite as often but are much easier to rank well for. Set out your keyword strategy to match what you're doing on your website and with other social medi

Optimize Your Pinterest Username

On Pinterest you can choose a username that is a keyword. This will help a lot because if your username is a keyword for your niche, whenever someone inputs that term into the search bar, your Pinboards will come up in the search. You'll get a lot more followers without even trying if you put a keyword in as your username.

Create a Full Keyword-Rich About Section

Pinterest gives a generous-sized about section that you can use to fill with information, tell your story and use keywords within the text to do so. Don't keyword stuff or force it, but using keywords within the about section is a smart idea as it will help your customers to find you when they search for those keywords.

Create Optimized Pin Descriptions

One of the best ways to improve SEO is to make use of the description area for your pins. You have a pretty big space to work with. Make them readable, but also include relevant keywords and URLs when appropriate.

Always Link Back to Your Website

You can link each pin that you create back to your site and back to specific pages of your site. Always take advantage of this and make sure they don't always just go to the home page. Make pins link back to specific landing pages on your website that are relevant to the pin.

Watermark Your Images

No matter what you do, someone might take your picture and try to use it as their own. But you can watermark it with your logo and URL. Try to do so as unobtrusively as possible, but watermarking will help with SEO too.

Don't Forget the ALT Text on Images

When you upload an image, or put an image on your website, you have something called an ALT tag or text. This is an area where you should use keywords to describe the image. Don't just say "butterfly" – say something like "This is a picture of a monarch butterfly that I took using my Nikon D700." This type of ALT tag would be relevant to a pinboard devoted to photography.

Make Your Website the Home for All Images

Everything starts and ends with your website. When you want to create pins and pinboards, first create a blog post with the image, infographic and post, then pin to the board from your website so that visitors always link back to your site.

Create Themes for Pinboards

Don't just randomly post pins. Instead, create themed pinboards where the theme fits with your niche and is a keyword for your niche. This gives you more areas to include keywords and more in-depth information about your niche for your followers. You can think of pinboards as categories like you have on your blog if that helps.

Use Appropriate Hashtags

Like most social media today, Pinterest also supports hashtags. Use them well and they will pay off. Really give thought to what the hashtags should be and how they relate to your niche before including them.

Re-Pin Items That Carry Your Keywords

Look up your keywords, maybe one or two a day, and re-pin other people's pinboards and pins that carry your keywords. In addition, follow them and their followers – just a few each day to help build your own following and interaction.

Using these tips to make your Pinterest Search Engine Optimization friendly will go far in helping you make the most of Pinterest as a marketing channel for your business.

Get more followers on Pinterest

Getting more followers on Pinterest isn't much different from getting followers on any other social media platform. You must be a contributing part of the community on a regular and ongoing basis, ask for people to follow you and follow them back.

Add a Pinterest Tab on Facebook

You can easily add a tab on your Facebook page in order to encourage people to follow you on Pinterest. When you create the new tab, be sure to point it out and announce it to your Facebook likes.

Add a Follow Pin to Your Blog

Your blog and website should also have a follow me button for Pinterest. If you use WordPress there are many plugins available to make this a simple and almost automatic thing to do.

Connect with Your Friends

When you join Pinterest you get the option to invite the friends their system can find, using your email address book to determine who might be your friend.

Cross Promote Your Social Media

Using your email mailing list and other social media accounts, be sure to share your different social media accounts with easy share, like and follow buttons.

Comment on Popular Pinboards

When you comment on pinboards, everyone who sees your comment can follow you on Pinterest. If you comment, just say something intelligent and don't spam by asking people to follow you. Really communicate with others without "selling".

Post Original Content Regularly

Don't add 100 updates all at once; instead create them and then schedule them to go out periodically. This way you show up with something new often. And the more often you show up with something new, the more chances you have of people following you.

Repin Other People's Content Often

When someone has content that you like and that you find useful, repin it. The activity is going to show up to more people and then you'll have more of a chance to get new followers.

Use Keywords Wisely

Keywords are important because that's how people find you when they want to find certain types of pins. Add keywords in descriptions, board names, and anyplace you can to get more viewers.

Getting more followers on Pinterest will help increase the buzz about your business, as well as help bring more traffic to your website and blog. Plus, you may also gain email subscribers if you organize your pinboards in such a way that makes viewers curious about what else you have to offer. Build your followers, like your boards slowly and steadily, and you'll get a lot further and be more successful than if you do it too quickly.

Creating Business Boards for Pinterest

Pinterest is an online pin board, when you open a Pinterest account you'll be given server boards to help you get started. Each board has a theme, such as "Products I Love" or "Books worth Reading." But if you are using Pinterest for business, you will need to create boards that are relevant to your business, its message and offerings.

Creating boards is a simple process, on your home screen, just click "Add" and then click "Create a Board." From there you can name your board, select a category and dictate who can pin to the board.

Here are some tips for using Pinterest boards for business.

- Give some thought into your board names and don't select the first name that comes to mind. An interesting name will engage visitors and entice them to look at your board, and board names with targeted keywords will help with search engine optimization. Combine these two elements to come up with the most effective board names for your business.

- Choose an appropriate category, the categories are pretty straightforward, so this shouldn't be too difficult, the most important thing is to remember to actually choose one. If you create a new board as you're making a pin, you are not asked to choose a category, and you may not remember to go back and do it later. Then your board will not show up for users when they browse the site by category, and you could miss out on visitors so always place your boards in categories.

- Always add a description, because this is also often forgotten or neglected, but it's a great opportunity to create interest and including a few keywords phrases sure helps with SEO.

- Rearrange your boards as you need to, you can put your boards in any order you like, so place those that you want to feature first. If you have lots of boards, remember that those that are above the fold will always get more visits than those that visitors must scroll down to see.

- Choose your board covers wisely, each board has one photo that is featured as its cover. You can change the cover at any time by hovering over the board and clicking "Edit Board Cover." From there you can choose any photo from the board. I suggest you select one that will make visitors want to see more, it's also a good idea to change them from time to time so that from the outside they appear fresh.

- Create boards that will engage people, think about what you can do for Pinterest users, not what they can do for you. Themes that are useful or entertaining will bring in the most visitors. Instead of just creating a glorified sales catalog or advertisement, create boards that feature information or advice that is relevant to your market. Make them smile, laugh, and think and forget trying to close sales, this will happen automatically if you engage your visitors.

It's impossible to have a great Pinterest presence without actually having great boards. Concentrate on coming up with fun, attractive or helpful themes, and your audience will eagerly await your pins and you'll pretty soon be a Pinterest rock star.

No matter what social media platform you use, you should spend the time required to craft the best possible profile that you can, this holds true on Pinterest and everywhere else. Try and craft it in a businesslike manner and focussed on your target audience, because even though you are promoting yourself and your business story, ultimately everything is about your customers and not you.

Business Profile Name

When choosing your Pinterest profile name, you may want to choose your actual business name, or you might want to use a keyword rich profile name. That decision is up to you and depends on how you intend to use your Pinterest account. If you do use your business name, you can include keyword descriptors in the description of the business.

A Great Description of Your Business

Using keywords that your audience might look up, describe your business and how you plan to use Pinterest in the business and solve your customers problems. Let your audience know why they might want to follow your boards and get to know you better.

Use A Great Pinterest Profile Picture

For your business account your profile picture can be your logo or a good picture of you. It depends on what type of business you have. If it's a freelance business, a picture of you is a great idea, if your business is larger and there are more people employed, using your logo is a good idea.

Website Information

Don't forget to include your website URL and include some information about what they'll find on your website if they visit it.

Other Social Media Accounts

Integrate your other social media account into your Pinterest profile by providing the URLs of them within your profile.

Descriptive Board Names

Start five to six different boards with descriptive keyword rich names that your target audience will understand and potentially search for.

Keyword Rich Description for Boards

Don't forget to always fill out the description of every pinboard so that it will help your audience find them, when searching.

Utilize Appropriate Board Cover Photos

Always remember to select the right cover photo for your boards, resize it as instructed so that it shows the whole picture without the need to click on it.

Organize Your Boards

Remember that when people look at any account they see the top boards, so put your most important boards at the top. You might even want to rearrange them occasionally in order to be sure all your boards are seen.

If you get all of the information to put on your Pinterest business account ready prior to starting your account, you should be able to set this up in just a couple of hours. If you've already started an account, you can go back and change things. Even the name of your business if you chose poorly the first time.

To fill out your Pinterest account faster, put up at least five or six different categories of boards for your business account and keep it up dated on a regular basis if you want results. You can add to the boards, reorganize them, and other things to keep them up to date.

Social media is a way for businesses to build relationships with their customers, increase brand awareness, market their products and to also provide excellent customer service. Social media is the new word of mouth marketing, in its word of mouth marketing on steroids.

When I started networking or word of mouth marketing, it was typically done behind closed doors. Now you can see how your brand gets known via the best word-of-mouth marketing ever invented, social media. Along with that wonderful window into your marketplace comes the need to provide customer service on each social media channel, as this goes hand in hand with word of mouth marketing.

Using LinkedIn

LinkedIn is the world's largest public accessible database of business professionals in the world and utilizing it to get more customers is essentially what LinkedIn is designed to do. Unfortunately you cannot just create any old profile if you actually complete one fully, disappear for extended periods and expect new customers to magically appear and come your way. Whereas what you need to do is create an awesome profile and actively seek to engage others, as LinkedIn is about building relationships.

Create an Awesome Profile

Don't waste space within your LinkedIn profile, use every space offered to make the most of your profile. Include a professional image, along with your professional work history. Make your profile work for the jobs you want, not the jobs you have had already.

Use Bullets and Whitespace

It's hard to read large blocks of text online without using bullets and whitespace to give the eye a break and even draw it in. Even in your LinkedIn profile summary section it's important not to write a whole bunch of text all together, as people will simply not read it.

Include Examples of Your Work

LinkedIn offers you the ability to upload examples of your work that other social media websites do not. Even if you cannot include actual samples due to non-disclosure agreements, create some examples specifically for your portfolio that can be shared. People want to see what you can do, and you have an unprecedented opportunity to really impress them.

Add Video

Most online professional social media platforms don't offer such an organized means of sharing your work, allowing a lot of information to get lost. With LinkedIn you can easily add in video, some great examples to use are a video introduction, recorded presentations and speeches, and how-to videos. These will show your expertise in a way that resonates with your audience on LinkedIn.

Ask for Recommendations

LinkedIn offers an easy way to ask for recommendations. Make sure you take advantage of it but go a step further by personalizing your requests rather than sending a mass message that is the same to everyone. You'll get a better response and they'll appreciate your having taken the time to remind them about what you did, the results of what you did, and how you remember them.

Contribute Content to LinkedIn

You can become a LinkedIn publisher by clicking the little paperclip on the right side of the status bar. This enables you to create longer articles than a normal status update. Use this to contribute professional articles with images. Try not use it as a way to blog, but instead as a way to demonstrate your knowledge and expertise.

Share Important Industry Updates

Show your expertise by sharing important information about your industry from trusted sources. Make comments and share your opinion on what you share, to add to and start a discussion about the information that you're sharing, even if you disagree with what you're sharing, say so with evidence-based research as to why.

Engage with Other Members

When trying to build relationships and make connections, it's imperative that you also contribute to other people's conversations, questions, and messages. This will help you showcase your expertise but also your willingness to communicate with others, making you stand out from the pack and get noticed.

Find Out Who Looks at Your LinkedIn Profile

You can find out who has seen your profile and if they look like someone who needs the services that you provide. Be sure to send them an InMail, or if they have provided enough information, contact them outside of LinkedIn to see if they need the services or products you're offering.

You really can find lots more customers on LinkedIn if you work at it. You can improve your professional image, develop your reputation as an expert, and win new customers using your LinkedIn profile.

Missed Opportunities on LinkedIn

If you're in business you should be utilizing LinkedIn, as it's a very effective way to find and connect with new customers, partners, suppliers and connections. Think of LinkedIn as the largest and most up-to-date database of businesses and business professionals in the world, because that is what it is and LinkedIn gives you free access to. However as with most things, people tend to make mistakes and this leads to missed opportunities, so let's have a look at a few common LinkedIn profile mistakes.

Not Using a Professional Image

LinkedIn is the most professional of the social media platforms and it needs to be treated in a professional manner. This means that you need to utilize a professional looking photograph of you and not an image of you with your children, the dog or cat, leave that for Facebook. Similarly people connect and want relationships with people so don't use your company Logo, use a great headshot the represents you.

Not Using the Summary Area

Use the summary area properly, this means using good grammar, punctuation and symbols to separate the information you provide. Reading on a computer screen is difficult and requires a lot of white space and separation, especially as people tend to scan content. The summary area is a great place to explain either what you do, or what you want to do.

Not Using the Headline Area Correctly

To best utilize the headline area, notice how many characters shown and how the profile looks to other users. Use the pipe symbol " | " to separate words within the headline. Also notice that on the headline area near your picture, your current position as well as some of your past positions are shown. If these positions have nothing to do with what you want to do, change how it is seen.

Not Filling Out Your Profile Completely

There may be some areas of the profile that you may do not want to fill in. That's okay, but do fill it out as completely as possible with accurate information, until you have an all-star rating. There is no reason to hide who you are on LinkedIn, that's the whole point of LinkedIn.

If you're looking to improve your career you should treat it like a resume. Build the resume for the job you want, not the job you have. Alternatively you can use your profile as a business development type area to network with others on that basis.

Not Asking Personally for Recommendations

You should aim to have recommendations that show up on your profile, but do not make the mistake of connecting to everyone and sending a mass message asking for recommendations. Take the time to personally invite each person to provide you a personalized recommendation by reminding them of your skills and what you did for them or by asking them to do it themselves based on what they know about you.

Not Editing for Typos and Grammar

One of worst things that can happen is to have a profile that has a lot of poor grammar and typos, have someone you trust look at your profile to see if they notice anything that needs correcting. Ideally you want to ask a few people to do this, as sometimes things are easily missed.

Not Creating a Personalized URL

LinkedIn provides a link that is just a few random letters and numbers, it's important that you personalize it with your name, what you do, or your business name.

Not Submitting Samples of Your Work

Your profile allows you to include samples of your work. If you have no samples right now, create some. If you say you're a speaker and presenter, upload a video showcasing this.

By maximizing your LinkedIn profile to attract potential connections, get more clients, and even find your next job will work if you take it seriously, fill it out completely, use professional language, a great photograph, and the right keywords and that you stay focused on what you want to achieve from LinkedIn.

I know lots of LinkedIn experts and most of these people are extremely knowledgeable about LinkedIn and how it works. They can help you setup your profile, teach you how to use the search feature and how to get introduced to potential people of interest. Sounds great doesn't it and I am sure you can benefit from using such services, you might even find a new job or locate a few new clients.

Let's look at this for a minute:

- **Complete All Star Profile**: You complete your profile: include appropriate keywords that the LinkedIn search engine can associate with your profile.

- **Search and Advanced Search**: Learning to use the search feature is great if you ever use it.

- **Connecting with People**: Learning how to connect with someone you don't know, how to get introduced, how to always write a personal connection request, etc.

- **Interacting**: You'll learn how to join the groups your prospects frequent and to interact with them, and get to know them.

- **Sales and Prospecting**: Occasionally someone you know might ask you for something and you'll learn how to make contact (email, telephone, etc.); with supposed warm contacts.

- **Tips and Tricks**: You'll also learn how to use updates, how to make posts, how often, plus each expert tends to have a bag of tricks that they'll teach you.

The reason I don't use LinkedIn this way isn't because I don't know how, it's because I gave up making cold calls many years ago and I don't plan on doing the LinkedIn equivalent of Inmails, messages and cold calling connections although to be fair some of these might be classed as warm contacts depending on the relationship you have with them, this is what I consider to be outbound marketing and not the best use of my time or resources.

The way I use LinkedIn sees my first level connections grow by around a hundred per week, I also have over ten thousand followers on LinkedIn and this number grows each week and best of all I receive enquiries for my services each and every week, normally ranging between three and ten per week and these are people contacting me, not me contacting them with requests. These figures are in my experience exceptional and are testament to the Inbound marketing tactics that I use on LinkedIn… and yes, you did hear correctly I employ inbound marketing tactics on LinkedIn, in fact I prefer to call it content marketing and that's something I'm exceptional at.

I have been doing profile marketing for a long time - long before Google existed and long before the term content marketing was coined and became popular.

The basis of my marketing on LinkedIn revolves around Long Form Publishing a feature LinkedIn introduced to all English speakers and which has revolutionized how LinkedIn should be used in my opinion.

Each day I publish at least one new article on LinkedIn, all I basically do is take an old article of a few months from my blog and repurpose it on LinkedIn, as it is published first on my own website and indexed by Google, Google understands that I am the authority website and LinkedIn is the secondary. As I understand my sales funnel and my target audience and the different audience personas at each stage of my sales funnel, the content is aimed specifically at one persona and has one goal, my aim is to drive my authority upwards and to slowly move each audience member along my sales funnel using nothing but the content I produce.

Think about that for a moment, I am using content that I am first using on my blog on LinkedIn to enable my target audience to find me, as each piece of content is search engine optimized. Once they find me I engage them through content, using a call to action these people are invited to follow me, to connect with me or to place an inquiry directly with me. The results I am generating prove that this almost scientific type approach to content marketing work exceptionally well on LinkedIn.

If you want to generate some real LinkedIn results perhaps you look at long form publishing, if you're looking for a LinkedIn trainer, expert, etc… to help you set up either look in the list below or contact me directly… and if you're a LinkedIn consultant, trainer, expert or whatever you call yourself please consider adding your details below so that people interested in getting help, setting things up can contact you directly.

Facebook Advertising

If you're looking for more customers and are interested in advertising, Facebook advertising on Facebook is one option that you should seriously consider. Facebook advertising is extraordinary in its ability to select a very specific target audience, monitor the effectiveness of your advertisements, and modify the advertisements to try and improve your conversion rates. To help you maximize your results from Facebook Advertising, try taking these few key steps.

- Begin With a Clear Goal. Two of the most common goals would be to generate sales directly from the ad or to increase awareness of your business while building a contact list for future marketing efforts. Everything about your ad should be constructed with your primary goal in mind.

- Choose the Geographic Area. Does your business only serve your local area? Do you sell products that can easily be shipped anywhere in the world? For either of these cases or anything in between, you can tailor the regions where your ads will appear to match your needs.

- Customize Your Ad for The Demographic You Wish to Reach. Because of the information Facebook collects about its users, you can define the advertisement's target market based on age, gender, location, interests, or several other criteria. Combining those criteria allows you to be specific when you construct your ad for that target.

- Direct Your Ad to Existing Contacts. Upload a customer or contact email list. Any of the people on that list that are also Facebook members will receive your ad.

- Set Your Budget. You can choose to run ads continuously or for a particular period, and you can select how much you are willing to pay. Budgets are set as a maximum daily expenditure or total expenditure over the duration of the campaign.

6   Use Images. Images receive far more interest and generate higher response rates than text-only ads. Consider creating multiple ads with different images to examine their relative effectiveness.

7   Use Facebook Ad Manager. Ad Manager accumulates metrics on responses to your ads and presents them in comparison to goals established when the campaign was initiated. Using the information available, you can alter the campaign, changing the budget or target market or even completely re-creating the ad. A big plus – Facebook Ad Manager is available as a smartphone app.

8   Use Conversion Tracking. With Conversion Tracking, you place JavaScript code on your website that tracks visitors' actions. That JavaScript sends info to Facebook, where it is compared with their record of prospects that looked at or clicked on your ad. Among other things, you can determine how many people viewed your website or made a purchase after seeing your Facebook ad.

9   Boost your posts. Boosting a post is a different type of advertising. Boosting a post causes it to appear higher in the News Feed of the ad recipients, thus raising the likelihood that it will be seen. You can have any post boosted, increasing its exposure.

10 Always include a Call to Action. Salespeople know the axiom "Always ask for the sale." Professional salespeople do not present information to prospects and hope they will choose to buy. They offer the information and ask the prospect to act, to make the purchase. You need to do that in every advertisement you create. Depending upon your desired response, include buttons or links asking the reader to respond. "Click Here to Buy," "Like This Page," or "Click Here to Receive My Newsletter" for example.

Follow these few tips when creating your Facebook advertisements and watch, monitor and adjust until you get the response you want.

Facebook Pages

One of the best way to market your business on Facebook is through a Facebook Page dedicated to that business. However, your personal Facebook Profile presents some marketing opportunities of its own. Utilizing your personal profile starts with personal relationships to build business relationships.

- Let your friends know about your business. Make posts that specifically focus on the business. You can put a lot of information in one post, but it would be more effective to go through a number of posts, spread out over time, with each having a tidbit of information. The multiple posts increase the chances that any particular friend will see the post.

- When friends share your posts about your business and their friends Like or Comment on them, consider sending Friend Requests to those new contacts. If they accept your Friend Request, you have new friends that will be seeing your posts regularly.

- Use your ability to select whether each post can be seen by only Friends or by the Public to expand your ability to use your personal profile to interact with the Public.

- You should also Allow Follows. When you Allow Follows to your personal profile, you don't have to accept individuals as Friends to for them to see all of your public updates. You also won't have your news feed cluttered with the updates of all of your followers.

- Even personal posts can connect to your business. Your business is a major part of your life, so it is natural that some of your personal posts will involve things that are happening in your business. Keep those posts personal for your friends, but don't overlook the opportunities to promote your business subtly at the same time.

- Don't hesitate to create posts to your personal profile that are solely ads for your business. This is an effective place to do that, because your friends already trust you. You have to build that trust in new contacts. Keep it in balance, though. Even your friends will lose interest in your Facebook posts if they are about nothing but your business.

- Whatever the nature of post, if there is any connection to your business, include business contact info or a link to your website.

- Always work to find ways to include a "Call to Action." Whatever you are doing to promote your business on Facebook, asking the reader to take some action that will strengthen their connection to your business is essential. Some possibilities are links to take them to your website or Facebook Page, or to sign up for your mailing list to receive an informative report or other information. Any response to a Call to Action gives you more information about the prospect and presents an additional opportunity to make them a customer.

- Use images intensively. A company logo, a photo of your place of business, or a photo of employees involved in some public service activity – any image like this draws more attention and gets more responses than text alone. Include text with, or even within, the image to further enhance its ability to create interest.

- Any professional certification or award is a subject of personal pride, but don't overlook it as an opportunity to promote your business.

When marketing your business on Facebook, you have an entire suite of tools available. Don't overlook the opportunities presented by your personal profile, especially as it shows your personally and exactly who you are.

Expanding on Social Media Opportunities

As business owners you most likely understand the value of utilizing social media to market your business. You have most likely created a Facebook page, a LinkedIn profile, my own favorite a Twitter account, all with the hope of expanding your marketing efforts. What you might not realize however that there are many more benefits of using social media than just marketing. With proper use and deployment of social media, any business can do all of the following and probably more.

Social Media Allows You to Find Employees and Contractors

Need to find a new employee fast? Use social media to help. Simply create a detailed job description and post it on your social media accounts. Ask your friends and followers to share it, and they will as it is potentially helping someone they know. It's also much more likely that the person(s) who answer a call like this, will be more compatible than using say a huge impersonal job type board.

Create more Sales

Many people confuse sales with marketing, thinking they are the same thing but they're not. Marketing is best described as increasing your reach so that you can generate more leads, sales is the conversion of leads into customers and then into repeat customers, both are intertwined but different. Social media can help to increase sales outside of your marketing efforts just because your clients might share with others what they bought (social proof). And if they like what you are talking about on social media, they might like to buy from you more.

Reward Customers

Provide discounts, pins, stickers, badges, games and more for your customers using social media to "check in" or communicate with you via social media. People love getting free things and they love collecting things, so take advantage of that by using social media to encourage more interaction with your customers and between your customers.

Brand your Business

As a business owner it's important that you spend the time to brand your business across all of your chosen social media accounts, as honest, relevant, customer focused and even generous. Try to monitor as best you can how your audience, customers and employees view your business via the interactions on your social media channels. Listen to your customers, let me repeat that listen to your customers and be perceived as a business that does. Demonstrate these things as often as possible as a way to brand your business on social media.

Motivate Employees

Recognizing good employees on social media is a great way to encourage employees, if you have an employee of the month program, don't just post it on the notice in the canteen; paste it all over social media. They'll share it with their family and friends and it might even be picked up by the local media, encouraging employees to even greater highs.

Speed up Communication

You can set up private closed groups on Facebook that only employees can see, it's a great way to speed up communication between employees and to build your own company community. Encourage your workers to follow each other and encourage each other and publicly acknowledge them.

Easy Project Collaboration

Another potential use for private Facebook groups is easy project collaboration. In Facebook groups you can upload documents and communicate easily in one spot about various projects, without ever having to have a face to face meeting, but still be able to keep excellent records of the events and ideas as they unfold.

By being actively involved with social media, your business can increase employee happiness and satisfaction as well as consumer perception. Utilize social media to form a connection with your community and your employees. Any business can be an integral part of your community in every way that it can, be it a government department, social, business, or even a charity. Pick and choose to stay aligned with your purpose and target market, but do get involved however do remember it is better to be active and to work well on one or two social media platforms rather than be on them all and work poorly.

The key to marketing success is getting an effective promotional message about your company in front of large numbers of potential customers. Facebook Groups is an excellent tool for making large numbers of people aware of your business, your products or services, and your message. For dramatic increases in the visibility of your company, you might:

- Search Groups for interests that you would expect your customers to have. For example, if you sell camping gear, search for groups using keywords like camping, hunting, or outdoors. You will find many groups that are relevant to your business. Don't hesitate to join them all.

- Post to those groups, and do it often. Posting more than once a day is helpful. More posts increase the likelihood that any individual member of the group will see your post. Since you may be joining dozens of groups, unique posts for each group would be impractical. Create posts that can be used across the whole range of groups you have joined.

- Use images in your posts. Images get far more interest and response than simple text posts.

- Include links to your website or a call to action ("Click for more information" for example) with images. Your first goal is to build exposure, and a large fan base is evidence of that growing exposure. You want the group's members to go to your Facebook page, where they will find more information about you, your company and your products.

- Create some item that can be emailed at regular intervals. Whether in posts to the group or on your Facebook page, you should have a call to action – Sign Up For My Newsletter, for example. When visitors sign up for that newsletter you grow your email list, which can become an entirely separate marketing tool.

- Do not post only ads to the groups. Also create posts that actually provide value, whether entertainment or information, to the reader. You want to build a relationship with the reader that makes them more inclined to trust your business..

- Whether posting ads or informative or entertaining posts, address problems that your product or service will solve for them. It doesn't have to be a blatant cry for their business. Just making people think about the problem and creating an awareness that you can help contributes to the relationship.

- Use giveaways to encourage visits to your Facebook page. Giveaways don't have to be costly. An informative report that addresses visitors' interests or can cost you nothing to put together and increase your Facebook fan's interest in your business.

- In all of your efforts, keep in mind that your success is dependent upon building a relationship with the individuals in the group and with the visitors to your Facebook page. Whether they are a few dozen or a few thousand, gear your campaigns to individuals, not groups.

- Be Honest. Sure, that's your intention, but don't let promotional puffery slip over into false statements. Assume that the reader will at some point become aware that a claim or a promise was false. When they reach that awareness, all of your effort toward building a relationship is at risk. It is much better to promise less and deliver on every promise.

For an explosive growth in your Facebook Page's fan base, and a corresponding growth in sales, there is no more effective single tool than Facebook Groups. Make them a consistent element of your marketing plan.

In the process of looking for ways to increase sales, you have probably realized the root question in any marketing campaign is "How do I get information about my business in front of people?" Before you even decide on the content of your marketing message, you have to know that people will see it.

That means knowing where people will be.

Facebook is where people are, with over 1.3 billion active users. And on any given day, 48% of them log on. You can target your desired demographic in that enormous audience by creating a Facebook Page, so let's look at some ways to use a Facebook Page to market your business.

- Create a page. That is your starting point, so don't put it off. It is quick, easy and free. You can have a Facebook page for your business up and running in less than an hour, and you can refine it as frequently as you wish.

- Add a cover and a profile picture. Some graphic representation of your business (a photo or your logo, for instance) will create brand awareness for that image. People that have visited your Facebook Page will have a connection with all of the information they have received there whenever they see that it.

- Add a "Call to Action." On the Cover area of your page, set up a call to action. Use it. Also use Call to Action buttons or links in your posts and in ads you create. Responses to a Call to Action build your fan base and create alternative ways to market to those fans.

- Add a description of your business. This is the first place visitors will see information about the nature of your business. You have two places for descriptions – a short one (155 characters) and a long one. Use both.

- Add contact information to encourage prospects to find you. Add your address, telephone number and website URL to your page. Some businesses will use a Facebook Page in lieu of a website. If you have a website, though, a leading function of the Facebook Page will be to drive traffic to it.

- Post on your personal Facebook Profile to acquaint your friends with your Facebook Page. Ask them to Like your Facebook Page. (Another Call to Action!

- Through your Page, connect with Facebook Groups that have the interests that you expect your customers will have. There is no better way to increase your business' exposure quickly.

- Start posting and do it often. You increase the chances of any given Facebook fan seeing your post when you post at least two or three times per day.

- Do not post only ads on your page. Your main reason for creating the page is to increase your business, but an advantage of Facebook over most marketing tools is the ability to build a relationship with prospects. Give them reasons to like you. Give them entertaining and informative posts, as well as ads.

- Allow others to post to your Page. This provides an opportunity for two-way communication with prospects – another step in building a relationship rather than merely dispensing ads. There are options available to provide monitoring so you can protect your page from inappropriate language, for example.

Start with your Facebook Page to grow brand awareness and respect from visitors to your Page. This one tool can start an exponential growth spurt.

Perception is everything, especially online and as a business owner this means your online presence is perhaps your most important method to market your business both locally and internationally if you wish. It doesn't matter if your business is online or not, it has to be represented online and today we're going to discuss the importance of social media and how a business should establish its identity online.

Ensure that Your Brand Matches Throughout

Every social media platform has its own personally, its ways of doing this and presenting your information, in a similar fashion your business brand is always your business brand. This means that no matter what social platform someone encounters your brand on, it should basically be the same just adjusted slightly to fit in with the personality of the social media platform. But it's not changed all that much because you want your audience to recognize you and interact with you.

Keep Your Profile Updated and Complete

Social media platforms are constantly evolving with new features being added and modifications being made. This means that your profile that you worked so hard to complete fully might not be complete tomorrow, so ensure it is up-to-date by checking it often, updating the things that have changed, and adding in new information as the social media platform creates new ways for you to share.

Content is the Key to Success

One of the major ways to get social media to work for you is to actually get involved and post regular posts and updates. This obviously takes content and even though it's fine to use curated content (other peoples content) don't just share this, always share some of your own original content to maximize results and to drive people into your sales funnel. You also want to post updates multiple times per day and not just once a day, social media is crowed and people's attention is always on the latest and greatest posts so that blog post you want to share, share it twice in a day instead of just once.

Become the Best You can be on One or Two Platforms

Unless you have a small army of staff you don't want to be on every social media platform. I've had to close down my company Facebook page simply because I can do two platforms really well, but I can't do three. For me Twitter and LinkedIn are the two platforms I have chosen, I'm passionate about them and more importantly my audience is there.

If you can afford to outsource your social media workload or have staff members to spare then by all means try and conquer every social media platform. But if it's just you, take it easy and become the best you can be on one or two platforms, if you're like me you'll get much better results.

Develop Content Specific for Each Social Media Platform

You don't want to rehash the exact same content in the exact same words on each social media network. For example, when you share a blog post you wrote promoting your content marketing services or your latest and greatest product, you want to share it with a special blurb for each different networks, so that you reach both audiences.

Engage with Others

Social media isn't just about promoting your content, in fact it's all about engaging with your audience and that means engaging with them. Talk to people, answer questions and share your knowledge as you engage with them, you'll be amazed at the response.

Even if you automate most of your social media marketing, it's imperative that you spend time interacting personally with your audience, this is what works and what turns an audience into fans... automation is great but it only goes so far, people like to interact with people, not machines.

Share Other People's Updates

When someone you follow or know shares something your audience will find interesting, share it. The people you share and

155

congratulate and interact with, will do the same for you. Plus, it's another form of content that can help establish expertise.

Join Groups

Most social media platforms have some forms of groups that you can join. Even Pinterest has group pin boards that you can join. Joining these, then interacting with other members of the group, is a great way to network and develop relationships.

Every business should have a social media presence, it complements a website perfectly and helps drive people to it, whilst reaching a potential new audience and developing deeper more personal relationships. Use the social media to promote what you put on your website, as well as to stimulate sales of your products and services and watch those conversion rates improve.

I have to admit that my own social media accounts are not focused on Facebook, this is predominantly because I have a limited amount of time and that I find other platforms of more use to me in reaching my target audience. That doesn't mean that I don't value Facebook or understand how it works, it simply means that I prefer to run two social media accounts extremely well rather than three or more less effectively.

Anyway let's talk about Facebook because to many online marketers it's a real boon as it's not only the largest of the social media platforms, it's also the most addictive and you can achieve an awful for little or no cost, apart from your time that is.

Set Up a Business Page

Every business should have its own business page as this offers you some added features that personal accounts lack at the moment. To set up a business page on Facebook, you first need a personal page. But once you do have that, its easy set up your business page. The business page enables you to promote your business actively while a personal page is not supposed to be used for that. It's also free to set up and the ability to schedule posts and get access to Facebook stats makes this extremely worthwhile.

Set Up a Community

A Facebook community is very useful in terms of being able to discuss things with your customers, or potential future customers. You can easily set up a community in the same way you set up the business page, simply choose "community." A community has more communication ability between your likes and followers than a business page.

Set Up a Private Group

A private group is a great way to run a small or even large mastermind group without having to invest in the technology yourself. You can make them private and even secret. If you have a secret group, you'll have to actively recruit people to join; you can even charge people money to join if your group offers enough value to warrant it.

Promote a Post

On your business pages you'll have the capability to post things and you'll get a button that offers you to "promote" the post, which means you can advertise your post. You can bid a certain amount that you wish to pay but where Facebook comes into its own is in its ability to allow you to choose your audience. Not only that but you can really narrow down your focus so that it only appears to a very select few, this is pure genius and it's what makes Facebook advertising one of, if not the most effective.

Run a PPC Advertizing Campaign

Even without a business page you can create advertisements via your personal page on Facebook. It's wonderful because you can narrow down your target audience in ways that you may not have realized that you could. You can target with age, sex, location, groups and affiliations. It doesn't get much more niched down than that and nothing else comes close to allowing this sort of focus.

Join Groups and Communities

A great way to market your business on Facebook is to join other peoples groups that attract your target audience. Then, simply help others, don't try and sell just be yourself and help and don't have an agenda other than helping and getting involved. Build your reputation by helping and then let your reputation speak for you.

Comment on Pages, Groups and Communities

When it comes to marketing on Facebook, a good use of your time is to make smart, intelligent and useful comments on posts that the owner of the page or group post, as well as being helpful to others who post. The aim is to be seen to be helpful and in the end a resource to others, so that people automatically turn to you for help and advice.

Share and Like

If you want people to share what you are doing, be sure to share and like what they are doing, human nature is simple, and we help those that help us. Facebook has some amazing communities when it comes down to it. You'll find competitors sharing each other's work and actively help one another, instead of bashing each other to bits. In fact I use Facebook to chat with many of my competitors although they are actually friends now, as we all help one another.

Using Facebook to market your business is an excellent way to market your business online. You can do so many things including contests, sharing images, memes, videos, blog posts, and more. If your target audience is on Facebook, and you have a liking for the platform you should jump right in and get started using Facebook to market your business today. But, be warned, you need to follow Facebook's terms of service in order to continue as you do with any social media platform or you risk losing your account.

Becoming a social media manager is a dream job for many, however just like every other small business you will be faced by one of the biggest challenges, how to market your skills to potential clients. As you should already know the ins and outs of marketing through social media, you should have the insight needed to be able to reach out and engage your social media audience, turning some of these from interested observers into engaged prospects and then into customers and raving fans. However you'll soon realize that social media alone isn't enough.

To really succeed as a social media manager you need to be able to reach out beyond those already using social media to find those businesses who don't have the time, the knowledge or the confidence to market themselves through social media even though they will have heard of the importance of social media marketing.

Here are a few ways you can market your social media selling services to potential clients.

Get a Great Website

It doesn't matter if you're the best social media selling expert around your website should still be the center of your marketing universe, simply because it is the one thing that you own and control. Facebook, LinkedIn, Twitter and the others can and do change, your website doesn't unless it's something you want. Your website needs to reflect your social media knowledge, you want people to arrive at your website and go, wow this person knows all about social media. It isn't enough to simply tell people how to do something, you actually have to show them and practice what you preach.

Additionally, you will want to include content such as that which is comprised of current stats and data from some of the projects you are working on, this data is unique to you, using it gives you a massive point of difference. You might also want to include comparisons between your work and your competitors, simply illustrate how you're existing and future service offerings (work), will and will continue to be better than those of your competitors. You often see this from of comparison given as a table, with ticks next to each service, which generally means the company with the most ticks offers the more comprehensive range of services.

You should also include testimonials and feedback from clients, statistical data from any metrics that you track, before and after project milestones, etc., not of course forgetting that you should actually incorporate social media within your website, show your audience your playground and just how good you are.

Blog about it.

Every business website needs to incorporate a blog, without one it's just a static often dead website. Once your blog is up and running, just blog about the techniques that you have found to be the most effective, also include those areas that you are perhaps not quite as good as, because simply by writing about them you'll actually learn more about them. Explain where and how you use these techniques, showcase the results and what can be learned from them, from a business perspective. These posts will form your most valuable authority content.

You should also address all of those questions and concerns that have ever been raised with you. Simply blog about them, answer each question as best as you can in one blog post because blog posts work best when you answer one question with one blog post. By doing this you will address all of the concerns, wants and desires of your audience and while you are doing it, you will have attracted an audience to your blog via basic search engine optimization and of course you will be promoting your blog via those social media channels you know so well.

Blog about techniques you have found to be highly effective as well as those you feel are lacking. Explain where and how you used them, what the results show and how it can directly impact a business.

Stay on top of your game.

We all live in a fast paced world and perhaps the online world is that fastest of all, social media selling is constantly changing. It's vital that you stay on top of new and emerging technologies that help you keep your clients' one step ahead of their competitors. Blogging about, talking about and showcasing new methods will show your audience that you are a forward thinking leader, always striving to be the best you can be.

Host a Webinars.

Webinars are a great way to market your social media management services, because unlike traditional selling you are selling to potentially hundreds / thousands at the same time. Webinars allow you to teach potential new customers why hiring a social media manager (you) is important and you'll showcase the value you bring backed up by real life facts and figures. Not only that but you will be able to answer any questions your webinar audience has, which everyone attending will be able to hear and this will also positively reinforce you as the expert in your field.

Simply invite prospective clients, anyone on your mailing list, and people via your social media channels. Consider partnering with complimentary business owners to co-host webinars, as you'll not only reach your audience but theirs too.

Once a webinar is over ensure you give your prospective new customers a strong call to action, because this is the time when they want what you have to offer, so tell them what you want them to do.

You should also post a recording of your webinar on to your website (blog) for all of those people that could not attend the live event. You can also use any of the questions asked as topics for future blog content as these questions and your answers are what are important to your audience.

Host a Live Event

Just like a webinar, consider hosting a live event, with the popularity of meetup.com it has never been easier to attract an audience, over and above those methods already mentioned. A live event is very similar to hosting a webinar except you get to meet people face to face which makes the whole event much more personal. When I started my business, I hosted a live event in our backyard, I attracted around twenty local business owners ran through my presentation, answered their questions and closed with a call to action. The clients we secured at this event formed the backbone of my initial business and without them I would not have succeeded.

Advertise.

Word of mouth marketing is perhaps the most powerful way of marketing, it empowers your existing clients and fans so that they introduce you to new potential clients. However, if you don't have many existing customers, fans, friends and family it can be really hard to get word of mouth often referred to as referral marketing to work for you.

In such circumstances you might want to consider advertising, both online and offline to raise awareness of your business in your chosen market. There are numerous places you can advertise online and as a social media manager you no doubt know of many, however don't forget that offline marketing can be cheaper (classified ads) and can potentially reach thousands. As an added benefit once you are advertising with a local newspaper, the chances of your next press release sparking interest improve.

Marketing is never easy, especially for a new business. My experience shows it works like this, the newer you are in business the more desperate you are to secure clients, the more out of your way you will go to please them, etc... however your potential clients subconsciously know this and no matter what you do, they are hesitant to trust you with their business. Your task is to keep going, to gain in confidence and to secure clients. As you gain more confidence in yourself and your business you will start to portray this in everything you do, subconsciously your prospects will know and you'll find it much easier to gain clients. All of those difficult questions won't be asked anymore and the awesome answers you had prepared will become blog posts and rarely used.

I was rambling a little there, marketing is never an easy task but it is crucial to your business success. Making that first connection with a prospect is where it all starts so make it count. It's that initial step that sets the scene and gives you the opportunity to turn all those prospective customers into paying ones.

Why Twitter Is Relevant and Useful for Entrepreneurs

Twitter is still a formidable social media outlet that small businesses should continue to use for the near and far future. There are many reasons for that, such as:

- **Twitter is still informative** – Compared to other social media platforms, it's still easier to find information about groups, causes, and businesses via Twitter search. Hashtags make it easy to compile the information, and important people are still having important conversations on Twitter.

- **You can engage with anyone** – Due to the way Twitter works, you can potentially connect with anyone whether you follow them or not, and vice versa. Due to the ease of sharing and the ease of tagging people, before you know it you could be in a conversation with someone famous or at least famous in your group.

- **It's very responsive** – Using Twitter on mobile devices is still easier than using other social media on mobile devices. There is still a lot you can't do with mobile on Facebook that you can do with Twitter.

- **Search is easier** – It's so easy to filter out the things you don't want to see. You can look at only tweets for a particular topic which makes finding trends fast and easy. You can easily study your audience and potential audience on Twitter.

- **Easier to grow your Network** – There is an unwritten rule in that if you follow someone they will follow you back, using this general principle you can grow your network of followers as large as you want.

- **Twitter Analytic** – I just love Twitter analytic (stats) these tell me which of my tweets are working and driving traffic and which aren't.

Due to these factors, it's important for small businesses to realize that Twitter is still a useful tool for engagement, research, and promotion. You just have to do it the right way, if you are having issues with getting results from Twitter, you're simply doing it wrong and chances are you're trying to make something work without putting the work in.

Don't Pass Up Everyday Opportunities

Tweet about what you're doing right now, and ask your employees and your contractors to do this as well. Make it relevant to your audience. For instance, if you're working on a new eBook, say so. "5000 words down on my new eBook!" is a great example of a tweet that will get attention of your audience, and likely some "congratulations tweets" too. What fabulous interaction, from just a simple update that you can capitalize on time and time again.

Your Twitter followers not only care about your day and what you're doing, enough to read your tweets and correspond about them, they'll also be happy if you share anything profound from other tweets of people who you follow. Sharing, commenting, and engaging are all important aspects of being on Twitter. Without those three things you won't be successful. So, ditch the automation, and use Twitter for all it's worth, because it is still very relevant in social media marketing today, in fact I believe every single business should be active on Twitter.

I don't hide the fact that I'm a massive fan of Twitter, whenever I am advising businesses on marketing I always ask, do you have a Twitter account? If they don't I always suggest that they get one, and fast. Twitter is the number one social media source for driving traffic to your website. Let me expand on that so that there are no doubts, Twitter drives more people to my website than any of the other social media platforms combined. At the time of writing I am generating approximately six thousand website visitors per month, and this figure is growing as my followers grow, this figure represents more than most businesses attract in a year.

When you get started with Twitter, one of the first things you want to do is build a following. However we're talking about Twitter marketing so you don't just want any audience, you want your own followers to be drawn from your target audience. Let's look at ways of doing this.

Perfect Your Twitter Profile

This holds true for all social media platforms, your profile is your main shop front and as such it's an essential element in ensuring the right people follow you. Click here to view my profile, I'm not saying mine is the best but it does work for me, once you have viewed mine, view industry influencers in your niche and simply take the best bits from each and incorporate them in your own profile, with your own twist of course. Use a good headshot, and use your main keyword phrase within your bio and don't pretend to be anything that you aren't, just be yourself.

Tweet Regularly

The average life of a tweet is roughly about eight minutes which means that you need to tweet regularly. Tweets are not like emails, they don't sit there until someone reads them, think of Twitter as a stream and your tweet as a boat floating down it, and if you turn away the tweet (boat) will float right past you without you ever knowing. This is how tweets work with your audience, they work only when your audience is tuned in and using twitter.

This means that you need to work out a solid tweeting schedule that works for you and that you can stick to, if you don't stick to it and tweet regularly people will soon forget about you. Use technology if you need to, to send out automated tweets for you and all you have to do is schedule them.

Grow your Account

There is an unwritten rule that if you follow someone that will follow you back, even today this still holds true for approximately 40 percent of the people you follow. This means that you need to follow as many people within your target audience each day, Twitter allows you to follow a maximum of 1000 people each day.

Simple math means that if you follow a thousand people per day and forty percent follow you back, when you have two thousand followers you will have around eight hundred of your own followers. This two thousand figure is a massive roadblock imposed by Twitter with the intention of stopping people spamming lots of people, however once you hit two thousand followers you are not allowed to follow any more people. That is until you have what twitter considers the appropriate amount of followers of your own, which happens to be 1819 followers. Twitter works by allowing you to follow the number of followers you have plus 10% which means that once you hit 1819 followers you can follow that many people plus 182 others (10%) which means you break the limit of being able to follow 2000 people, with 2001 being your new limit.

Sounds easy... well it is, all you have to do is un-follow the people that aren't following you, this allows you to grow your followers and break the Twitter barrier and then continue to grow while remaining within your ten percent limit. Does that sound like hard work, well there is technology available to make it easier, allowing you to see you isn't following you at a glance and then allowing you to click on each person to un-follow. Twitter terms forbid a fully automated system and although these exist if you get caught using one, you risk losing your Twitter account.

All you have to do now is rinse and repeat these follow, un-follow procedures until you have as many followers as you want, the secret however isn't to get as many as you can. But to focus on getting as many of your target audience to follow you as you can. This is the main reason that buying followers is a complete waste of time, the people that will follow you are not your target audience and you will never get any interaction from then, and as such they are pointless.

Engage with Your Followers

Now that you have as many followers as you want, you need to engage your audience. Even if your tweets are scheduled using something like HootSuite.com to help you manage your Twitter account (it helps manage more social media platforms), you still need to engage with your followers. This means that you have to look in your stream locate tweets from others that will be of interest to your audience and then simply retweet them. It's also worthwhile looking at your notifications tab and also mentions to see if people have sent you tweets, asked questions or left comments and if they have respond to them. This can take as little as 10 minutes each day but if you don't do it, you'll never engage your audience and they won't bother to engage with you. This action also helps you attract more followers because it makes you real and relevant.

Become a Resource to Others

The best part of engaging with your followers is to also become a resource center, this applies to all social media platforms. It works as simple as this, if you see something that you thing a particular user would like, or your while audience send them the link on Twitter. Your followers will appreciate it, and will love that you care enough to help them with no real benefit to yourself. By being active in discussions, sharing and linking to relevant content you will attract followers, it just seems to happen of its own this also happens offline if you regularly go networking.

Learn the Lingo

If you don't understand the lingo, the short cuts or the use of #hashtags then don't use them until you have learned how. #hashtags are one of the most useful things but they are also one of the most abused. To use them appropriately use hashtags that are relevant to the content you are sharing at that time and only use one or two anything else is just overkill. By properly using hashtags you allow others to find your content, you build trust and of course all those people that find your content will want to follow you.

Developing a large meaningful following on Twitter takes a bit of time, and especially if it's a large following but it is always worth it if you go about it the right way… see you all on Twitter.

Avoid These Social Media Mistakes

From my own personal experience I know that social media marketing is an excellent way to increase your businesses exposure and to generate website visitors, leads and money. However, there are also many common mistakes that people often make when engaging in social media marketing, if you find that you are making any of these, just remember it's never too late to fix your social media marketing and make it much more effective.

Not Engaging Your Audience

When your audience makes a comment on something, shares or asks a question, don't leave it too long to respond as this is an opportunity for real engagement with your audience. If you utilize a monitoring service or employ someone to monitor your social media profiles, have them inform you of ongoing conversations and opportunities for engagement. Or alternatively check yourself every few hours, the important thing is to engage and that engagement should be from you.

Poorly-Completed Profiles

I see this a lot especially on LinkedIn, incomplete profiles make your business look either sloppy, lazy or fake. If you want to be taken seriously and want to generate results, fill out your profile completely, include a good profile picture (of you on LinkedIn), your company logo/banner and information so that you can be easily contacted outside of social media, on your website or telephone for instance.

Not Focusing on Follower Quality

Some people make the mistake of focusing on the quantity of followers rather than the quality. You want to concern yourself with finding followers who are potential customers or who can refer to onward to potential customers. This is the reason that those people that buy followers are simply wasting their money, followers need to be real people that can potentially do your business some good.

Not Posting Regular, Relevant Updates

If you aren't active on social media posting things that resonate with your audience, then you're not going to get any real traction. If you plan to be successful with social media marketing it takes perseverance and patience, so post those updates often and regular and capture your audience's attention and then keep it.

Not Choosing Your Social Media Platforms Wisely

When I first started networking long before Facebook, LinkedIn and Twitter existed I was taught that you network in the places your customers go, This still holds true today in that you don't need to be on every single social media platform, instead simply be on the social media platforms your audience love.

I also believe that it's much, much better to be very active on one or two social media channels rather than weak on all of them. My own personal choice is LinkedIn and Twitter, I understand both of these, I have many followers and I know how to generate thousands of website visitors and multiple inquires weekly from each platform. Perhaps you can get similar results by focusing on your efforts on one or two social media channels rather than trying to master all of them.

Not Automating Some Tasks

My Twitter account is extremely active, it has a tweet being sent out roughly every fifteen to thirty minutes, these tweets are all automated which means that I have set it up once and I reap the benefit every single day. On top of this I also use one of the many social media monitoring tools which allows me to login and see who has replied to a tweet, or has sent me a message and how each tweet has performed. This then allows me to interact with my audience, reply to them and to really get down and personal with them and all it takes is ten to fifteen minutes two or three times per day. It's possible to automate posts to almost all social media channels just make sure when using such tools that you don't come across as too robotic.

Interacting Personally

Every chance you get, it's important to make spur-of-the-moment updates that are relevant to your business and your goals. This will make you look more real in the eyes of your followers and it also makes social media fun.

Not Personalizing Messages for the Channel

Each social media platform is different from the others, even if you audience is the same you should tailor your message to the platform so that you maximize audience engagement. For instance on LinkedIn I love to post full articles as I find that these really engage my audience and help establish me as a influencer, yet on Facebook I only post snippets that lead through to my blog. By personalizing your message for each channel you also come across as a professional and instead of sending the same message, potentially to the same audience members which make them feel spammed, you will come across as fresh and engaging even if it's the same news item being discussed.

Using social media to market your business is a proven technique to get more customers, make more sales, and increase your bottom line, but only if you avoid these common mistakes. Work on one social media platform at a time and make the improvements needed to get it back on the right track so that you make your **social media marketing** profitable for your business. Oh and remember you can check my Twitter and LinkedIn accounts account to see exactly what I am doing and see the successes I am experiencing.

Don't Let Social Media Consume or Control You

It seems as if everyone uses social media and as a business owner it makes perfect sense to use social media marketing to get the word out about your business, products and services. However you also need to understand that social media marketing has the potential to draw you in and become a major time waster and even worse still your customers can often see you doing this. If you want to ensure that social media is not controlling you at work, follow these tips.

Have a Plan of Action

If you fail to plan, you are going to waste an awful lot of time on social media so don't do anything without a plan, as this will help ensure social media marketing will work well for your business.

Create a Social Media Publication Calendar

Plan your posts ahead of time and schedule posts in accordance with what you specifically want to promote, making sure all of your updates have a purpose. If you have a calendar with pre-written posts, you can easily schedule them to work to meet your business goal.

Avoid Time Sucker Activities

It's way too easy to get suckered into yet another personality quiz or discussions about what one of your friends had for dinner, or perhaps you'll get suckered into playing some sort of game or commenting on some cute picture or a million and one other things. It's fine to do all of this, but do it after work is complete and you are on your own time clock.

Outsource Scheduling

Once you create a publication calendar that matches your promotions you can give the list of updates to someone else, your virtual assistance for example to schedule and monitor. However, don't make that an excuse not to engage personally and share your opinion.

Take Time to Comment and Engage

Even if you outsource parts of your social media marketing, be sure to personally comment and engage your followers so that they know you are a real person to trust and know you.

Do More of What Works

If you do something that works, do more of it and less of what isn't working for you. Monitor the metrics of everything that you do so that you are positive about what is working and what is not working, simple isn't it?

Each Post Needs a Reason for Being

Don't post something without a purpose. If you don't know why you are posting it, don't post it.

Don't Forget Your Call to Action

Everything you do should have a CTA. Whether it is to share, follow, or click, ensure clarity about what you want your audience members to do. If they know what you want them to do, they're more likely to do it.

Using social media correctly to market your business is an essential marketing technique today in the world of advertising and marketing. Social media marketing can be very effective and pretty inexpensive if you are careful not to waste time and effort on messing around and doing things that have no purpose.

Mimic the Experts

There are lots of successful social media experts, some much more successful than others but all of them know what it takes to make social media work for them and for you. Aside from making regular updates, relevant posts for their audience, and stand-out content, they make sure that they stay involved in each social media platform in a personal way.

Make Your Social Media Profiles Stand Out

Everything to do with social media is about getting noticed for the right reasons but luckily everything you need to know is on display, if you just look and learn. When completing your profile the best advice I can give anyone is to find some industry leaders in your industry or look at a few social media experts you respect and look at exactly how they have completed their own profiles. Study these profiles and learn from them, take the best bits from each and seek to improve them and you'll then understand what makes for a great profile on that social media channel. Each social media platform has its own personality and way of doing things, but your profile on each platform should resonate with your audience so that someone following you on more than one platform can instantly know you. It's also extremely important to fully complete your profile, which on LinkedIn for instance will give you an "all-star" rating.

Make the Right Connections

Once your profile is fully completed, it's time to connect with those industry influencers, movers and shakers. By connecting to social media influencers you will get more traction because if you are seen to connect with each other, have conversations and interact, all of their followers will see it and more importantly they will see you.

Make Your Business Pages Interactive and Informative

I used to push people towards having a business page on each social media platform and I still do provided your business is large enough. And if it is you should not skimp on making your pages represent your business and look awesome. Since the launch of LinkedIn long form publishing my view has changed as this brings so many benefits I advise all chief executives, business owners to utilize this as a great way to promote their businesses and their own profiles.

Share Relevant Industry Topics

If you want to quickly become a go-to expert, find or create relevant industry news and share it with your followers. Don't worry about giving it away, your competitors know it all already and by giving it away you'll move to a new, better level with your audience.

Join the Conversation

Don't just simply post articles and news, you have got to jump in and start interacting with your audience, this means entering comments, sharing your opinion and entering into conversations with others. Think of it as a social gathering and just jump right in and start talking and interacting, your audience will love it and you'll become more and more popular.

Learn to Use Hashtags

Hashtags help you and others organize and search for relevant content on social media. Always use the # before the word, use no punctuation, keep it as short as possible and use letters and numbers.

Advertise Strategically

One of the best places to advertise is on social media, it's a great way to get the word out about a new product or service. However, be strategic when running an advertisement so that you know exactly what you expect to achieve with it, before starting to advertise.

Use Sponsored Ads and Posts

When you have something important to get across to your audience, it's important to use sponsored ads where many eyes are on the post. Please keep an eye of your budget.

Hire an Experienced Copywriter

Content is king, this holds true for all social media platforms it's therefore beneficial at times to work with a copywriter who understands your business and your voice, to help you with many of the posts and get them right within the space needed.

Be Yourself When You Post

When you are in a discussion on social media, outside of representing your business you are also representing yourself. Be who you are, share your opinion so that your social media presence has a personality and never pretend to be something you are not, as you'll come across as fake and you'll never succeed.

ou don't have to reinvent the wheel when you get involved with social media marketing, simply follow the experts and watch and learn what they are doing and do it yourself. Focus on differentiating yourself and being a real person with a unique voice that represents your business and your audience will love you.

Google+ is #1 for Business
Google Plus Is The Most Important Social Media for Business

If I was to ask you to name the number one Internet Company, chances are you would say Google, because Google owns the largest share of the search engine traffic. This means that as a website owner, it's extremely important to pay attention to whatever Google is doing, including **Google Plus (+)**. <u>Google Plus seems to want to be Facebook, Twitter and Skype all rolled into one</u>. And it's succeeding. The reason you need to be involved, read that again the reason you need a *Google Plus* account is that Google Search is going to rank your website higher than they would someone else's who uses anther companies social media tools. This means that if you want your website to appear better than your competitors you had better start with a Google Plus account, because if your competitor doesn't have one your already ahead of the game.

Google Plus Aids Adwords
Linking the two together with social extensions is an important way to ensure that all your plus 1s are linked for search purposes. When your Google+ count shows up in search engines, users are more likely to click through.

Google Authorship
This is a very important way to claim any writing you've authored. It also influences click-through rates because the listing shows your picture, along with increasing page rank of such results.

Local Optimization

Search results are now very personal and take into consideration the location of a signed-in user, even if the searcher does not put their location in when searching for something. This is useful for local businesses but all business types can take advantage of local search.

Latest Activity

When you conduct a search for a product, service or brand, notice that on the right hand side of the search results you can see the most recent activity of that brand. This gives searchers a chance to see recent blog posts and other activity at a glance which will increase click-through rates.

YouTube

Now that YouTube is part of Google, anything you do on YouTube now shows up better in Google search results. Your Google+ profile picture shows up next to your YouTube profile, plus you can auto post YouTube videos to Google+ updates.

Using all the different features of Google Plus offers huge advantages to any online marketer who wants to take the time to learn about the features mentioned above. Google is constantly rolling out even more features which promise to benefit online and offline business owners even more. There are ways to improve page rank and search results using Google Plus that are spelled out in Google's Webmaster Tools. Your website is linked to Googles Webmaster Tools isn't it?

Because Google is the top search engine, owning over 65 percent of market share, it's important not to ignore the importance of the features Google puts out. Using Google Plus and all its features will benefit you much more than using similar features outside of the Google Plus platform.

That doesn't mean you should stop using other social media, but it does mean that much of your effort should stay with Google. **Recognizing the importance of Google+ and all the tools available for your**

business will ensure that you are using all the features that can enhance your online marketing efforts.

The Goooooooooogle+ Audience

Google+ is not the place to put advertisements and marketing information. Instead it's a place to get to know people, let them get to know you, and post the things that are interesting, informative, interactive and inspirational. You want people to see what you have to say, make you part of their circles and come to your Google Hangouts.

Use Buttons and Badges

There are several badge types and buttons that you can grab the code for to help people find you from other online properties, but there are also buttons and badges you can use within Google+ that can assist with people finding your Google Hangout and other activities. Follow the rules of Google badges and buttons for proper use.

Get Verified

Google allows you to verify your business, yourself and your profiles. Be sure to do the process. The extra steps are an excellent way to build trust with others. After all, your focus is on building an audience of followers who want to get to know you better. If you're not verifiably you, it won't work as well.

Post Enough

Google+ is not Twitter, or Facebook. You don't need a continuous stream of posts. Post things that are thoughtful, smart, informative and engaging two or three times a day unless one thing you post causes a lot of stir, in which case focus on that one for that day.

Identify and Engage Influencers

Use the tools that Google+ has developed such as Ripples, Search and Explore. When someone pluses up one of your posts, you can use the Explore link to find out more about them and Ripples to find out how far, and who else has shared your post, and who with. These are likely new people that you can add to your circles.

Add a Google+ Link to Your Website

Seems like a no-brainer but you must put your Google+ link on your website and other social media. Cross-promoting is the best way to get people to follow you because some people prefer one type of social media over another.

Interact with Others

Don't just plus things; also comment, discuss, and find ways to interact with others on Google. When you do that, they're likely to add you to their circles faster, building your following and an audience quickly.

Promote Other People's Posts

It's important that if you see a post someone made that fits your audiences, you comment on it and share it. Starting the sharing will help others want to do the same for the things you share.

Use Google Hangouts

You want to collaborate, communicate and discus with like-minded people on Google Hangouts. This is an excellent way to build a following and an audience who is ready to watch you and interact with you. Hold regular round table discussion with other colleagues live on Google Hangout so that the public can watch.

Google+ is very useful to help you get more traffic to your website, as well as help you accumulate a fast-growing group of followers who will interact with you. Yes, eventually they will find their way to your sales pages, and buy from you too. But, being more interested in building relationships on this social media platform is the best way to go about it.

Maximize Your Success

Every business should be using social media to promote their business, as it can be extremely lucrative if you know how to make the most of it. You need to remember that social media is not a short term commitment, it takes time and a long term commitment as well as realistic goals in mind to succeed.

Complete Your Profiles

Completely fill out your profiles, using keywords that your audience as well as search engines would most likely use to find you. Show your personality, link to your online real estate, and make sure people can connect with you easily. It's also a good idea to ensure all of your profiles on all of your social media accounts follow a similar theme so that people can recognize you, easily on each of them.

Post Quality Content

Get known for posting quality content, so take your time to consider whether the content you are thinking of posting is relevant, has quality components and will give your audience a reason to want to keep following you. By doing this, consistently your audience will grow and will look forward to all of your posts.

Play the Long Game

Social media marketing results don't happen overnight. It takes time, months normally of consistent and focussed activity to start to get the outcomes that you want. If you expect instant results, you're going to be disappointed, so understand that it takes time but the rewards are well worth it.

Engage Influencers

Use the search function on all social media networks to find movers and shakers within your industry so that you can engage with them. Getting their attention in a good way will help increase your influence too. In fact if you want to be seen as an influencer in your own right simply interview other influencers, by doing so they will help promote their own interviews that you carried out, and as such they will promote you and simply by being associated with them your own influence increases.

Avoid Time Wasting

When you get on social media it's very tempting to start looking at posts after all many of them are interesting, talk to your friends and family, play online games, and pretend you're working. This is time wasting, and lots of business people waste a lot of time, do what you have to do on social media, take ten minutes for yourself and then get off and get on with your day… otherwise you'll spend hours doing nothing.

What Goes Around Comes Around

If you want people to comment and share your information, be sure that you do the same for them. The best course of action is if someone markets to your same audience but is not direct competition, try working together to promote each other.

Pay for Promotion

When you are trying to get a more likes, followers or newsletter sign-ups, if you have the budget it's a good idea to pay for promotion. On Facebook you can pay to promote particular posts, or run a pay-per-click ad relatively inexpensively.

Add Real Value

Don't just like and tweet things without adding something to the conversation, the more value you can add to social media discussions, the more people will want to get to know you and follow, friend and like you, oh and never be afraid to share your opinion, it's what makes you unique.

Using social media to promote your business is a great way to get more visitors to your website and make more sales, I know I generate in excess of five thousand new visitors each and every month. But, you have to be committed to your audience, give them what they want and take the time to do what it takes to reach your goals. Avoid pretending to "work" on social media while you're really just socializing, I see this way too often. Set specific realistic goals, develop tactics to reach these goals, and you will be successful.

Writing Posts Customers Respond To

One of the things to do on social media is to write articles, this content is what helps keep your social media active and your audience engaged. I have found however that it's extremely helpful to have a strategy so that you can supercharge your social media interactions. For many this means that your social media strategy should involve building your email list or in getting your social media audience to your website so that they can become customers.

Understand Your Customers

As always you need to know who your target audience is, so that you can understand how best to engage them. Let me give you an example, if you post articles of a certain politic view point and your audience has a different one to yours, another example could be the use of comedy in your posts, some people might be insulted and others could respond exceptionally well. The point is this, once you know who your audience is you can ensure the content you use is targeted to them.

Watch Your Competition

Social media is great in allowing you to check out what your competition is doing in regard to social media posts. You don't want to copy what your competition is doing, instead try to observe which of their social media posts are generating results, which aren't and then use this information to make your own perform better.

Know the Purpose of the Post

What do you want your audience members to do when they read the post? Do you want them to click through to your website read more? Do you want them to like, follow and share? You need to understand what you want them to do in order to get them to do it.

Use Suitable Image

People respond better to posts containing relevant images on social media, you can make can make memes and infographic using free software such as Canva.com. A nice image, watermarked with a relevant quote works wonders in a post or even on its own on some social media platforms.

Write Some Blurb that Gets People's Attention

When you share something on social media write something interesting about it, share your opinion, and tell people what you want then to do with it.

Link to your Blog

Don't just post content without linking to your blog, give your audience a chance to read more and build your email list and website followers up at the same time.

Ask Your Audience to Share

Never forget to ask your audience to share your posts. You can also invite them to take memes and infographics off your website to share directly as they see fit. Just set up a new page that lists all the watermarked images that your audience can share and then invite your audience to do so.

Answer Comments

People are generally less likely to leave comments than they were a few years ago, so don't just ignore the interaction that is happening on your social media pages. Always respond, and add comments to the discussion. Answer questions, and be kind. Even if someone is rude, and upsets you and don't forget if it is really bad you can delete it, and then move on without rising to the bait. Unfortunately people do this on purpose to get a reaction, these are called trolls… if you don't rise to the bait they will move on.

Writing social media posts that get a discussion going and inspire people to share and interact is an art form. You'll need to try different tactics to see what works with your particular audience. But, always make sure to always have a call to action on anything that you post so that your audience knows what to do. Remember that your goal is to get them on to your email list so that you can market to them over the long term or to visit your website to become a customer.

Instagram Your Way to Millions in Sales

Instagram launched in October 2010, Instagram is an online photo sharing service that has taken the world by storm. By its third month of existence, it had gained its first million registered users. Today, it boasts in excess of 300 million regular monthly users with hundreds of millions of photos uploaded. The company was purchased by Facebook for around a billion dollars in cash and stock in 2012.

There are plenty of other photo sharing services online, many of which have existed long before Instagram, so what makes Instagram different?

Instagram Filters

Instagram makes it easy for users to enhance and manipulate their photos by using filters, each filter employs preset adjustments to color, tint and brightness to give the picture a unique and professional look.

Portability

The Instagram app is available for free for iPhones and Android phones / devices. Once you've downloaded it, you can take a picture, choose a filter, add a caption if you like and instantly post it to your Instagram account. Think about that for a minute, it's free, quick and extremely easy to do all of those things with your phone.

Social features

Instagram is actually as much about social networking as it is about photo sharing, users can follow one anothers photo streams, allowing their photos to show up in their feeds as they are posted. They can "like" and comment on photos and they can also easily share their Instagram photos on other social networks like Facebook and Twitter.

Photo Maps

Instagram users can choose to display their photos on a Photo Map, which organizes the photographs according to where they were taken and displays them on a map. Photos can be added to the map when they are uploaded or at a time afterwards. You can also remove photos from your map or turn off photo mapping altogether should you wish.

The popularity of Instagram has made it a useful tool for businesses, marketers can share photographs of products, services and events with their followers, enticing them to interact with and learn more about their businesses. They can also set images to post to their other social media accounts, giving them an easy way to add content and additional opportunities to engage their audience on other platforms.

The last decade or so has seen a massive rise in the popularity of social media and this has created a wealth of opportunities for business owners. Twitter especially makes it super simple, quick and easy to get your message out to your audience, wherever they may be. But the world of social media is constantly changing and evolving, so it's important to keep up with current trends. Relatively new networks such as Instagram which started in October 2010, offer even more opportunities for marketeers.

Basically Instagram is a photo sharing application that sits on your phone, but its social networking features are amongst the best, hence its popularity. This makes it a wonderful tool for businesses, and here are some of the most effective ways you can use Instagram for business.

Showcase Your Products

Instagram is a great place to promote your products, especially those with visual appeal. Some businesses use it, like a catalog simply posting numerous photographs of their products. This can be effective in some cases, but a better approach is to show your products being used, in action so to say. If you sell cosmetics, for example, you could post images of customers using and wearing your products. These types of photographs make it easy for the customer to visualize themselves using your products.

Show the results of your products.

Unfortunately not all products have great visual appeal, but perhaps they produce visible results. Weight loss products are an obvious example of this, where you could show before and after photographs. This can also work well for a number of other products, such as hair loss treatments or beauty makeovers.

Inject some personality into your marketing efforts.

Even those businesses that provide services or create products that are not what you would term "pretty" enough for Instagram can use the Instagram to their advantage by showcasing their human side. The truth is we're all interested in other people and what they do, so some simple photographs of you and your team in action will be interesting to many users, especially if they are accompanied by a fun or thought provoking caption. It's also good to show your business engaging in charitable work or helping out in the community. You could even post photos of your employees or clients along with brief profiles.

Entice others to help promote your business.

Photo contests are great for getting your business noticed on Instagram, simply come up with a theme, and ask users to post images using a unique hashtag. You can offer a prize for the winner or simply feature the best photos on your website. If you can't afford to run a contest, simply finding photos users have posted that include your products and giving them a mention can help encourage others to post similar photos.

Instagram offers businesses a simple way to promote themselves and their products. It doesn't require a large time commitment or even a great deal of marketing expertise, this is why you should give it a try.

Analyze Your Competitors

As business owners we're always looking to give out businesses a boost and one of the best ways to do this is to check out your business competitors. Your competition, even if you business is as popular as Google, can give you a lot of insights into your audience and how you can improve and make your business even more popular and profitable. One of the easiest ways to do this nowadays is to analyze your competitions social media efforts, let's see how.

Follow your Competitions Social Media Activities on All Social Media Platforms

Look and try to understand how they are using each social media platform to give information to their audience, how they engage them, and how they get more followers. Does it appear that they are using automation software?

Sign Up for your Competitions Email List

Email lists are a really good way to check out your competition and see how they're using their email in conjunction with social media to market their products and services.

Read your Competitions Blog Often

Set up their blog on RSS feed so that you can keep track of the type of information they're disseminating to their audience. Do they ask their audience to share blog posts? Do they make it easy to share? Are they having success doing this? What are they doing that you aren't? Can you do it better?

What Do They Share Using Social Media?

What does their goal seem to be using social media? Do they try to lead you back to their email list, blog, website, other social media accounts, or something else?

How Do They Get People to Like or Follow Them?

Do your competitions social media marketing activities include offering incentives to their audience to like or follow them on multiple social media accounts? If so, are they giving new or the same information on each account?

How Often Do They Send Out Updates?

Track how often your competition sends out updates on each social media platform.

Track What Time Your Competition Sends Updates

What time is the most common time that your competition sends out updates on each social media platform?

What Is the Reaction of the Audience?

Is the audience engaging with your competition based on their updates? And how does the timing of each update affect this? Are your competition generating the best engagement due to updates being sent at the perfect time to reach their audience.

As you ask these questions, you will need to keep track of the answers. Some good ways to do this are:

Create a Spreadsheet – Enter the information you collect into a spreadsheet in order to keep track of the questions you have about how each of your competition uses social media.

Use Evernote – This is a great way to keep track of different things that you would like to try that your competition is doing. Make a note of it, and then put it into practice on your own.

Write a Report – Taking each of your competition separately, write a report with the information so that you can easily look at it for future reference.

Tracking your **competitions social media efforts** and how well they are doing, as well as how your audience responds to the competition, will help you know what to do more of in your own social media marketing efforts and will often give you a competitive advantage.

When businesses write copy for the numerous different media platforms, it's important to take into consideration the mood of the social media network as well as your target audience. The standards for website copy, email copy, and social media copy are all different and there are things you should take into consideration before you write the copy. Not only that, you don't simply want to put the same copy up everywhere, you want to be innovative and fresh on each platform, if you can. **Here are a few things you should consider when developing your own social media content strategy plan.**

What Platform Rules Exist?

Each platform has its own rules that you should keep in mind before you create the copy for that medium.

Should Your Content Be Short or Long?

Each social media platform requires different lengths of content. As you know, with Twitter, you only have 140 characters to get your point across. With Facebook you have a bit more space, and with Linkedin you can post whole articles. On your website blog and every single business website should have a blog, you technically have unlimited space. So consider which social media you're writing for before you write the copy and tailor it.

Which Subset of Your Audience Is Here?

You should know that every person who is a member of your target audience, is not connected to you via every one of your social media network. Some will be on Twitter, some on Facebook and some will only want to read your website blog. It's up to them, and something you should think about because the choice is with the reader not the business owner. Ideally you can study which subset of your audience is following you on each social media network so you can focus the copy more toward them.

Is the Platform Buttoned-Up (Liked LinkedIn) or More Free Like Twitter?

Some platforms are more serious and professional than others. That means that sharing that picture of the cat hung up in the blinds might

188

not be a good idea on LinkedIn, whereas sharing it on Facebook might be fine if you can relate it somehow to your business.

Should You Use #Hashtags or Keywords?

Even Facebook has got with the practice of using hashtags, but is it appropriate to use them on every platform? Probably not. Using them too much may show that you're not that creative after all.

Is the Platform Visually Based?

Yes, it's true that Twitter is trying to be more visual, as is Facebook. But, Pinterest and Instagram still lead the charge on being visual. Those two platforms would not do well with just a text-based update. You should consider that prior to creating the content.

What Are Your Social Media Content Strategy Objectives?

What is the point of your update or share? Do you know what you are hoping to achieve? Do you have a well thought out, specific, numbers-driven objective in which you can measure results? If you don't how will you know if it's a success?

Should You Include a CTA?

You should always include a Call To Action (CTA), but how you do it on each social media network is what's important. What type of CTA would tick off your audience, or would get you kicked out of the social media network? Avoid those and find out what works for you.

Is Your Copy Sharable?

A really important factor for social media copy is whether or not your copy is shareable. Shorter, visually oriented, relatable content is better to post on social media when you want it to be shared, and for most businesses that's exactly what you want to reach the largest audience.

Creating copy for social media is different from writing keyword rich articles, just like writing blog posts is different from writing for

Linkedin. As you create your social media content strategy, these differences must be apparent to you in order to achieve success on each platform.

Turn Facebook Fans into Paying Customers

Turning Facebook Fans into Paying Customers should be the aim of every business that utilizes Facebook, after all businesses are here to make money. So How do you convert fans into customers so that you can capitalize on your social media marketing? To most businesses this means a constant stream of sales messages which in my experience seldom convert fans into customers, however it isn't as difficult as many would think, here are a few different ways to maximize the potential of your social media following.

Offer a Free Product If They Like Your Page

Everyone likes free stuff and this is a common practice when it comes to Facebook. Offer your customers something free if they like your page, such as promotional material like a sticker or anything that relates to your business. This builds trust and trust builds sales.

Give a Discount to your Fans

You want to reward your fans for keeping in touch with your page, so give them something special. Discounts that are exclusive to the people who like your page make your fans feel that they're getting something that isn't available to everyone, which motivates them to buy.

Give Them an Inside Look

No one wants to think of a business as a faceless entity. Give people an inside look into your operation and the people behind it. Showcasing the fact that your business and its employees are human will help people feel more connected to you.

Get Testimonials from Customers

When it comes to promoting a business, there's no stronger way to do it than by word of mouth. Facebook pages have an option which allows your customers to leave reviews on your page. Make sure to implement this because a few positive reviews could help you see a big increase in your customer base.

Hold a Contest

Contests are always a good way to get people involved. Get creative with it. You need referrals, so ask people to refer their friends to your page and give the person who refers the most people some sort of reward.

Get People to Interact

A Facebook page that is just constantly talking about the business side of things can get monotonous. Don't be afraid to go off topic from time to time and get personal with people. Start conversations and get people talking. The more they interact with you, the more they will trust your brand.

Build an Email List

Social media marketing is a great way to promote your business but it can also be used as a way to incorporate other forms of marketing such as an email list. Encourage people to sign up for your email list by promising them deals which will be exclusive to members of the list.

Create Content They Can Share

Your Facebook fans can be your secret weapon when it comes to promoting your business. Using them to promote your business for you is a great way to get new customers. Be sure to create content that your fans can share in order to attract new ones.

Promote Events

Don't be afraid to get face to face with people. Organizing an event for your business or becoming a part of an event which is already taking place is a great way to get to know people. Use your Facebook as a way to meet people in real life by encouraging them to attend an event which you might also be attending.

When it comes to promoting yourself on Facebook, there are plenty of ways to do it. All of the methods above are great ways to create loyalty between your fans and your business. There's guaranteed to be something in this list that gets you results, so try these few ideas out and see the results for yourself.

Do you Know What To Post on FaceBook?

Get Guaranteed Results with These Suggestions

Facebook is without a doubt the king of social media; it's the most popular social networking website in the world, by a long, long way. In the past ten years it's managed to acquire billions of users, who seem at times to be addicted to the platform. This means from a business perspective that business owner, especially those that sell to consumers (B2C) needs to take note, they need to have an active Facebook page and you need to know what to post on Facebook so that it will help engage your audience and generate results.

Because let's face it, social networking is all about interaction, and if you can't get people to interact with your posts, you're almost certainly doing something wrong. Let's take a look at what types of Facebook posts that are guaranteed to get people involved and remember once you know what to post on Facebook, all you have to do is to do it regularly to maximize results.

Like or Comment

The Internet is a very visual medium nowadays and Facebook is an extremely visual social network and one way to use this to your advantage is to post a picture. The next step would be to put two pictures together, either side by side or one on top of the other and ask people to "like" if they prefer "picture a" or to comment if they prefer "picture b".

Ask an Open Ended Question

Open ended questions are one of the easiest ways to drive engagement on Facebook. Asking people what their favorite movie, band or website is could generate a lot of engagement depending on how many people are willing to answer.

Looking for Advice

People generally like to help others, so reaching out for help is a great way to get people to engage with your Facebook page. Asking people what the best way to complete a task such as cooking a food item, building something, training a pet or any other situation that would require input from other people is a great way to drive traffic.

Caption Contest

Finding a picture that looks like it's trying to say something funny is always a great time to hold a caption contest. Simply post the picture, ask people to add a caption in the comments and if the picture is good enough you should be getting massive amounts of comments in no time.

Like If You Do This

This post is almost too simple, Facebook users love pictures, so posting a picture of an activity or something people commonly enjoy and asking them to "like" the post if they enjoy it as well will certainly help you. A great example is posting a picture of ice cream and asking people to "like" the picture if they enjoy ice cream too. Honestly, though, who doesn't love ice cream?

Nostalgia Posts

Every generation is different and making people feel nostalgic is a great way to engage users. Questions such as "remember when you had to rewind a video tape to watch a movie?" could be a big hit with the right crowd.

What Would You Do?

We as people like to think about what we would do in different situations, asking people what they would do in certain situations is a great way to get some answers. Questions such as, "What would you do if you had 40 million dollars?" could end up getting you a lot of answers.

Fill in the Blank

Fill in the blank posts are also a pretty easy way to get people engaged. Asking someone to fill in the blank in sentences such as "my favorite food is (blank)" is another great way to get people to interact.

Name Something without the Letter (Blank) in It

Surely you've seen these types of posts before. Someone posts a status or picture asking you to name a fruit or vegetable without the letter "a" in its name. This is a fun way to keep people involved and almost always gets the type of reaction you're looking for.

Post a Picture

It can't be emphasized enough that Facebook users love photos. A great way to get people involved is to have them post a photo of their own. Post a status asking people to post a picture of their favorite vacation spot in the comments and watch how many responses you get.

Recommendations

Need a new website to visit? How about a new book to read or movie to watch? A great way to get people involved is to ask for recommendations and you might actually end up finding something you like.

Yes or No?

It might seem simple but yes or no questions are an easy way to get people talking. Even the simplest question such as asking people if they like pizza and telling them to respond with yes or no could work like a charm.

As you can see by the examples above, Facebook is a highly interactive social media website. You therefore need to constantly engage people to keep them interested in your page and if you use some of the examples above you should get plenty of people talking about you. Go on, give it a try, **now that you know what to post on Facebook you'll be amazed at the results**.

Build a Huge Following on Facebook

I'm not the biggest fan of Facebook, I know there are many social media experts that swear by it, but I much prefer Twitter... however that doesn't mean I don't know my stuff as far as Facebook is concerned, so let's help build you an active Facebook following.

Here are three of the most effective tricks for building a following on Facebook:

Post Relevant and Informative Content

It is important to post content about your business and products in addition to other relevant and engaging content. Local businesses can engage Facebook fans with news and information about their town or community. Current events are a great example of localized Facebook content that readers want to hear about.

Being informative will keep users returning to your Facebook Page and can also lead to your page being shared by your fans (hint, hint – do this). Whether your business is local or not, posting links to articles and tutorials is an effective way to include informative content and it also helps with your search engine optimization. You can post information from other websites or create your own content and brand it with your business name to build name recognition and increase brand awareness.

Ask Engaging Questions Often

Asking questions is a fantastic way to generate discussions on your Facebook Page, especially if you ask leading question. The answers your fans provide may give you insights into what your customers actually want, worry about and ideas about how to improve your current service or product offerings. There are some very specific types of questions that can lead to increased engagement and participation on your page.

Yes or no questions are very simple and can be quickly answered by Facebook users. Two great yes or no questions to ask users are if they have signed up to your newsletter or visited your website. These types of questions create awareness of the rest of your business, are quick and easy to answer, and are engaging at the same time.

You can also use polls to ask questions about customer preferences and interest. Facebook makes this really easy by visiting https://apps.facebook.com/my-polls/. While products and services are one subject for a poll, you can also have ones about current events or other topics related to your business. You can even have a weekly poll so that users will know to return to your page on a regular basis. As with any methods for increasing your following, the trick is to make it fun and users will come back frequently.

Have Contests

People love winning prizes and contests, especially if there are free products or a discount involved. By asking readers to like the content on your page or tweet your page to enter the contest, you can dramatically increase your following. When one of your readers likes or tweets your page, all their friends will see that. People are much more likely to like pages based on the recommendations of their friends and colleagues. In addition, you will build more brand awareness as your name is seen in more places on Facebook.

Building an active following on Facebook may take some time, but it is an essential part of every business's social media marketing plan. The key is to be engaging and post content consistently so that your followers have a reason to visit and interact.

4 Top Ways to Make Money on Facebook

Have you heard about Facebook, it's the most popular social media website in the world with millions of people hang out their daily? With all of these people hanging around and with the way social media works there has to be a way for people to make money doesn't there? And of course there is, that is one of the reasons Facebook is so successful because people also go there to make money.

When trying to work out an idea to make money on Facebook it can be as simple as looking at what others are doing and then simply figuring out how to do it better. Creating a page to determine what people want and developing a plan of action to deliver the service or product is another good money making idea.

Selling Products on Facebook

It's possible with Facebook apps to turn pages on Facebook into online stores, fans of yours can buy products directly from your Facebook pages. You can use the services of websites such as Lujure.com to create iframes that simply mirror your existing websites within Facebook pages and its surprising easy to do.

You can also post articles and links to separate items in your online store, and if you don't have your own online store you could consider drop-shipping products so that you are not responsible for stocking physical merchandise. With drop-shipping you make the sale and deal with the financial and the drop-shipping company deals with the delivery and fulfillment part.

Driving Traffic to Paid Content

Facebook pages can also be used to drive traffic to landing pages that often sell e-books and webinars. Often you will find people posting snippets of articles that link back to your website to get fans to visit your website. I personally do this on a daily basis and have the whole thing automated but you can easily replicate it by simply cutting and pasting in your url to the status update on Facebook, it will automatically pull content from your website to make it super easy. Many successful marketers also use this technique to link to an optin page for building their mailing list (the money is always in the list). You can then follow up with fans via email and build another avenue for an ongoing relationship.

Affiliate Marketing

Building a Facebook page around a specific interest is an effective technique used by affiliate marketers. Affiliate marketers can post links to relevant services or products they feel will be helpful to their fans. Cost per click campaigns can also be promoted using the same technique. Becoming an affiliate for a popular Facebook game is yet another way to make money promoting products on Facebook (I personally hate Facebook games). If you are considering affiliate marketing on Facebook, remember that Facebook is about sharing quality content first and promoting goods and services second. It is not about spamming fans and friends on a social site, this will get you banned and is not effective and can damage your reputation.

Facebook Apps

Developing apps for niche communities on Facebook can be very lucrative, both in terms of brand recognition and sales. If your app becomes popular on Facebook, your name gets known and more people will visit your website. Launching an affiliate program around your app would also help increase sales and quickly introduce customers to your product. Consider a need that is currently being unfulfilled in the market for a particular community. Then brainstorm ideas for the type of app you would like to create. You can outsource all the actual development to a freelance programmer which isn't as expensive as you might think, bringing Facebook Apps within the reach of anyone with a good idea and the commitment to make it work.

You do not have to reinvent the wheel to make money on Facebook. Consider the special communities you belong to and what you can promote to help that group. You may not even have to create a new product if you can find an established quality product or service to promote.

Scheduled Posts on Facebook – Yes or No?

Should You Use an Automated Facebook Poster?

Facebook marketing is all about interacting and connecting with current and potential customers. The challenging thing about using *Facebook* to promote your business is how much time it takes to engage and update on a regular basis. And we all know how distracting Facebook can me, one message and your off for ten minutes before you realize it, which is fine at home but not at work. Using tools to automate your Facebook marketing may be great for saving time and keeping things running smoothly in the office if it is done effectively.

Remembering proper <u>Facebook etiquette</u> when using autoposters is what can make them effective. Here are some general guidelines to help you save time and still engage customers with autoposters:

Create a Facebook marketing schedule.

The number one secret to most forms of content marketing is to schedule regular days and times to create status updates and stick to them. By scheduling regular updates throughout the week, you ensure your content is being published on a regular basis.

Check in to Facebook and respond.

The danger of autoposters is the ability to post content without ever engaging with your audience. Make sure you check in periodically during the week to answer any questions or comments you have received. It is a good idea to schedule this activity as well. Checking in on Mondays, Wednesdays, and Fridays is effective because these days are at the beginning, middle, and end of the week.

Double check all scheduled updates.

Be sure to double check your updates and make sure they are actually working and being posted. Technology is wonderful, but it does not always work the way we want it to and there is no excuse for not checking occasionally. Note whether or not scheduled updates have been posted on your Facebook wall when checking in to make sure everything is working as you intended.

Which Facebook Autoposters should you use?

You may be wondering which autoposters are the best to use for Facebook. Here are few reviews of popular autoposters:

Tweet Deck

Tweet Deck is owned by Twitter and is the ultimate tool for social media users. It has a robust amount of features including the ability to post updates on every major social media site (Facebook, Foursquare, Linkedin, Twitter, and MySpace). You can also view YouTube videos inside of the Tweet Deck platform. This is a very powerful dashboard that is easy to use and simplifies planning and centralizing all of your social media marketing. A common complaint about Tweet Deck is how much its desktop application can slow down your computer. They also have an app for the web, iPhones, and Android devices that make it very easy to use on the go. Users have the ability to drown out all of the social media noise and focus in on a specifics user's updates with its columns feature. Tweet Deck is available at www.TweetDeck.com

Hootsuite

If you are someone who is overwhelmed by too much activity or want a more simplistic tool for updating your Facebook Page, consider using Hootsuite. Hootsuite is a web-based application that is perfect for accessing social media accounts on your computer or mobile device. Hootsuite also allows you to manage accounts across multiple platforms and its built-in link shortener with analytics is a great feature for business users. Hootsuite also allows teams to collaborate and update company profiles. This tool may be the most ideal for larger businesses or businesses with an independent social media manager. The ability to select which social media accounts you want to link to and update may be ideal for users who are easily distracted while marketing online. Hootsuite is available at www.HootSuite.com

I personally use Hootsuite, however my setup is slightly different in that I have my blog set up to automatically post a new article each day, as this is published it is automatically shared around my social media network including Facebook with all the appropriate meta tags to ensure it is read correctly by Facebook. The every seven days the last four articles are automatically added to my newsletter and that is sent out automatically. I have a few more things happening especially with Twitter. I also use Hootsuite not to make posts, I use it so that I can login to one place and check all of my social media activity, so that I know what is happening.

Networked Blogs

Networked blogs is a wonderful platform for bloggers and blog readers alike. Blogggers can import their blogs into Facebook and blog readers can read their favorite blogs inside of Facebook's platform. Networked Blogs is another tool that allows social media users to centralize their web-based activities. Bloggers can also use a separate profile to promote their blog within the network. Networked blogs is great for people who want a tool that automatically updates their blog posts on Facebook.

It is definitely feasible to make your marketing efforts on Facebook easier with autoposters. Remembering basic Facebook etiquette in addition to using autoposters will help you expand your brand and create a more sustainable social media marketing plan. Research different autoposters to determine which one will be best for your business.

Get More Out of Your Social Media Marketing

Social media marketing is an extremely effective means of getting your message out about your products and services. However it's clear that most small business owners are not using social media marketing to its full advantage, most seem to think that social media marketing consists of sharing a few posts each day, but nothing could be further from the truth.

Complete Social Media Marketing Profiles.

Which of the social media networks you've determined are important enough to use for your business niche, it's extremely important that you create consistent and complete social media profiles. Include a professional headshot but please leave off of those cheesy chin holding poses, your aim is simply to look friendly and approachable not like the next super model. Keep the text of your profiles very similar in nature ensuring that one doesn't contradict the other, you want visitors to one to realize who you are immediately without having to guess and you don't want to confuse any that visit your other social media profiles.

Host Interesting Live Events

With services like Google Hangouts you can host live events such as a round table that is open to the public (open air) to watch, while your group discusses a hot topic within your niche. Another way to have a "live" event is to host a Twitter party (these are awesome if at times hard to keep up), or a Facebook party where everyone is allowed to post links to their own business or blogs for a specific amount of time. One way to do this is ask everyone to write a blog post about a specific topic and link to it within 24 hours, share and use a specific hashtag to promote the event.

Congratulate People & Get Involved

If you notice anyone having a special day on any of your social media accounts, be sure to congratulate them and wish them well. It's a good chance to make a connection with someone whom you're friends with or connected with that you don't necessarily know well and it's extremely easy to do, especially on Linkedin.

While a lot of people may be doing the same thing, people still like to be noticed for their achievements, accomplishments and special days. If you know their address, it's a good idea to also drop a card in the mail to make it even more special, just imagine how cool that would be.

Use Images in your Social Media Marketing

People who use social media prefer sharing and engaging with images over text. You should always include text with the images, though (for the sake of keywords), but creating images and memes using software like Pixlr.com is simple, fun and easy. You can do something as simple as a quote on a nice peaceful background and see a huge difference in the amount of engagement from your connections. And as much as I hate them, image spam abounds simply because it works and by image spam I mean images containing text such as "Answer this to prove your smart, write a word that starts with A and ends in E, you have 15 seconds" ... images of this nature attract lots of attention.

Use Social Media to Survey Your Audience

A great way to use social media to help get more engagement is to use it as a way to survey your audience to find out what they really need and want. But, don't give them too many choices. It should be more like when you get your child ready for school – give them two choices: this or that? Give your audience a choice between two different videos you can create or webinars that you will host. Then, ask them to vote or decide.

Capture Influencers' Attention

This can be tricky, but you want to find a way to call out influencers within your niche. If you can get a popular "guru" or authority within your niche to like, share, and connect with you, it's possible to quickly expand your audience. There are many different ways to do this, but one is to comment on their posts intelligently and share with your audience what the influencer is doing.

Finally, to get more out of social media marketing it's important to be truly engaged. Don't put everything on automatic. Don't hire someone to do your engagement for you, your customers and future customers want to engage and get to know you, not your social media marketing company. Make intelligent and purposeful comments, share freely, and you'll get more out of your social media marketing than if you automated it all or outsourced it all and best of all, you'll have fun doing it and the feedback you get could literally change your business for the better.

Social Proof & How to Get it

Social proof is a concept used in online marketing that businesses and individuals use to judge the trustworthiness and reliability of a person or business online, and that search engines such as Google also use to improve page rank for any given website. It's about engaging customers and potential customers and building trust and proving that you're reliable, honest and trust worthy.

We've all seen websites filled with testimonials and we all know that nobody actually believes these anymore, heck I could send to you a site now that will sell you video testimonials for just a few dollars… with Social Media proof, your trustworthiness is built up over time, it involves your customers and it's often their voices combined that give you true social proof.

Social Proof Starts with Being Social

If you're in business and you don't have any sort of social media account you're marketing in the dark ages and it's only a matter of time before your competitors are gaining more and more work from you, using social media and social proof in their marketing mix.

I believe every business should have accounts the likes of Google+, Twitter, Facebook, and Linkedin, they are free after all and you can't escape the importance of being social when it comes to online marketing. Friends of friends actually do care about what their friends and family are doing, saying and buying. The actions of the influencers in your life actually help determine the actions you might make.

Friends of a Feather…

Studies show that your closest friends influence not only your happiness but also your net worth. The saying that "birds of a feather, flock together" isn't really far off. This means that with the right connections on social media, if you can get the word out about your products and/or services to one of your most ideal clients, and they share, it will likely end up in the view of more of your ideal clients.

Word-of-Mouth Is Imperative

What's more is that most people trust word-of-mouth recommendations for products and services more than they trust any other type of marketing or advertising and most definitely more than they trust the testimonials on your website. If your best friend says she likes something, you can usually be sure you'll feel the same way. If someone you trust says they found value in something, you feel confident that you will too and chances are you'll check it out too.

Social Proof Takes Time and Effort

Developing and increasing your social proof happens through interaction on social media, blogging (does your business have a blog?), and participating in your community. It doesn't matter if your community is online or offline, I'm a member of my local Chamber of Commerce and various other business networking groups, because I value to social proof these groups give to me, all it takes is effort in getting to know those other businesses involved. Become an active participant and it will go far in creating the social proof that you need to be seen as a trustworthy source of information. The more people who start quoting you, the more people who friend you, follow you, and retweet your information, the more social proof you collect.

Use the Tools of the Trade

Tools like Google Authorship allow you to connect your articles and blog posts to your image in the search results. Plus creating branded social media URLs, along with a consistent image and profile will go far in ensuring that people know who you are. Once a person reads, enjoys, likes, shares and comments on something that you have written, they'll be more likely to see search results that your work appears in.

Before online marketing we already knew that customers were more likely to tell people if they had a bad experience or disliked a service than if the service was good. The tide has shifted somewhat in how people behave now that we have online communication and social media. Today, a person who likes something is likely to share with more than 1000 people over time due to the connections of others. Earning social proof is not something you can ignore if you want to market online successfully.

Why Isn't Facebook Enough?

Many small business owners have jumped on the Facebook Page bandwagon. Some are even abandoning the idea of having web pages and blogs in favor of a Facebook Page. It seems so much easier than the other options. However, this is a huge mistake. Facebook is not enough in the world of online marketing to make a difference. Here's why.

Your Online Presence Needs Many Entry Points

To attract your audience today you need several places in which they can find you. You need social media like Facebook, along with your website. Your website should be considered the main source for all your social media sharing. Your entire focus with social media should be to drive traffic, increase engagement, and improve the ranking of your website. Having only one point of entry into your business will leave out a lot of people.

Facebook Is Not Set Up to Provide Information in a Cohesive Way

If someone wants more information after seeing a post on Facebook, even if they go to your Facebook Page it is very hard to find information. Posts get hidden in the crowd. But, you can lead them to your website which can have information for your audience displayed in a cohesive way that can be used easily by them. They'll be able to contact you easier, and get more information on a website than they can on even the best made Facebook Page.

You Need to Build an Email List Too

While people may communicate with you via your Facebook Page, you also need to build an email list. You've heard it said that "the money is in the list" and it's not an exaggeration. Building an email list is an important factor in any business's success or failure. Communicating to your audience only through Facebook isn't enough; you must also build a targeted email list, capturing their information and sending up-to-date information to subscribers often. Email lists are still the best forms of direct marketing that exists.

You Don't Own Your Facebook Page

That's right; you don't own the Facebook Page and you can't back it up. You could be shut down for any reason on any given day. In addition, not every person who "likes" your page sees your updates. Facebook decides who sees your updates. You can pay for sponsored posts so that those who have already "liked" you can see your posts, but why would you do that? Facebook is an important part of online marketing, but it's not the only part of online marketing. In fact, it's not even the most important factor.

The most important factor in your online marketing efforts is your website. You control it, you own it, and you won't be wiped out just because someone else decides your content isn't good enough, or appropriate. You can't be wiped out without any warning like you can with social media like Facebook. Until and unless these facts change, you still need a self-hosted website to where you drive traffic from social media.

Leverage Social Media to Create More Buzz About Your Business

Social media is a great way to promote your business and create more buzz. It doesn't matter if you have a bricks and mortar business, or a completely online business. It also doesn't matter if you sell products or services. Using social media to create more buzz is something all business owners need to do. It's one of the best ways, that's really practically free, to get the word out about your business.

When you consider the fact that so many people are on social media (and not just on it; they keep it with them in the form of their mobile devices almost at all times), it becomes clear that you need to use social media to promote your business. At no other time in history has a business been able to be so close to their customers at all times.

Interact with Your Audience

The more you interact with your audience, the more likely they are to help you create buzz for items that you want to pass the word about. The audience won't feel as if they are being sold if you use social media regularly to interact with your audience. They will be more likely to share what you say if you're there all the time too.

Use Facebook for Events

It's free to use, so you might as well use Facebook events to spread the word about your events on social media. It's a great way to create buzz for an event because people can easily share it. It's also a great way to leverage free on social media. Nothing is better than free to promote something important to your business.

Use Google Hangouts On Air

If you have any events or grand message to send, a really good way to get buzz going is to have a Google Hangout On Air. This is a live event that you have some people join, and others watch it as it's happening live. You can do a roundtable event, discussing other important events to come, or sales, or whatever you want to. People will get to view you in action and share it with their friends too.

Tease Your Audience

Send out infographics, images, and more about your new product or service in advance of it being live. As you create parts of your product, share it. A book cover, a few paragraphs from your new book, some graphics and images that pique the interest of your audience will go far to create buzz and excitement about your new product or service.

Blog and Share

Most people don't think of blogging as social media, but the moment you open your comments up it is social. So blog about what's going on in your business and in your life if it fits, and open up those blogs to commenting. Ask for comments to get it started and respond to the comments to keep the discussion going.

Creating buzz about your business using social media is a quick way to get people talking about your business. It's as simple as setting up an account and getting started using the content you already have. Don't delay.

Marketing with YouTube

YouTube has only been online for a few short years, but it has quickly become one of the hottest destinations on the Internet. Once a little-used medium due to slow Internet connections, the widespread use of broadband has made online video a popular attraction. YouTube is one of the first sites to have been built around online video, and its ease of use and variety of videos has made it extremely popular.

Marketers were quick to catch on to the possibilities presented by YouTube. They began to create "viral videos", clips that were intended to draw interest and spark widespread distribution. YouTube's embed feature allows anyone to place videos on his blog or website, so by creating funny or informative videos, marketers could spread their message far and wide.

Any online marketer can harness the power of YouTube to promote his products, services and website. Here are some types of videos that tend to do well:

* Popular commercials – If you have a television commercial that has brought you lots of business, putting it on YouTube can get you more mileage out of it. And best of all, you don't have to pay for airtime.

* How-to videos – While some Internet users just want to be entertained, many of them come online looking for information. How-to videos allow them to see how something is done rather than just reading about it. Businesses capitalize on this by producing videos about how to do things that relate to their products or services.

* Video from special events – If you've held or participated in a conference, seminar or other special event, posting a video of it on YouTube could get you lots of traffic. So don't forget to take your video camera along!

* Funny videos – Lots of Internet users visit YouTube when they need a good laugh. If you can whip up a funny video that features your products or services, there's a good chance that it could be highly rated and go viral.

A frequent mistake of YouTube marketers is just uploading their video and hoping for the best. Here are some simple steps you can take to increase your video's chances of success.

* Take care to put your video in the right category, and make full use of tags. Add tags that describe your business and products, as well as the video's subject matter. This will help users find your video more easily.

* Write a good description that contains keywords that one might use to find your video. Also, be sure to include your site's URL in the description.

* Be sure to allow embedding, comments and ratings. Allowing others to embed your video will give it more exposure. Making it possible for them to comment will generate discussion, which is also good for your video's success. And allowing ratings could put you higher in YouTube's search rankings if people like your video.

YouTube is an invaluable marketing tool. It gives businesses the opportunity to use the popularity of online video to their advantage. Anyone can create a video with Windows Movie Maker and upload it to YouTube, so why not give it a try if you haven't already?

CHAPTER 13: VIDEOS

Common Mistakes that Video Creators Make

Video production is becoming easier and easier as technology gets cheaper and easier to use, however simply adding video to your content marketing mix, doesn't mean things will go as you planned. One of the best ways you can learn is to look at the mistakes other have made and learnt from, as this helps ensure you don't make the same mistakes, so here are nine common marketing video mistakes.

Making Your Video Too Promotional

When starting your content marketing journey you want to achieve the success you hear this form of marketing offers, you want to promote your business, your products and your services in some way, this applies to all forms of content you create including video. The problem however is that you are not making a commercial, if you did no one would want to watch it.

You're making a video that provides information, is educational or solves a problem of your audience, as well as providing positive reinforcement so that your audience want to buy from you. Just as with written content, include a call to action however make if less than 10 or 20 seconds at the end of the video, and make the rest of the video non-promotional.

Making Poor Quality Videos

Your video does not have to be of the highest quality, it's not a television production; if however you want it to potentially become popular with the potential of going viral then you should make the highest quality video that you're able to make. In addition, seek to make your videos better each time, as you learn more about lighting quality, sound and video editing.

Not Putting Your Video Where Your Audience Will See It

It might sound like a great idea to only put videos on your own website, due to branding concerns. But this is not going to build an audience very quickly, especially if your website is not that popular to start with. Even popular websites post videos to other places like YouTube, Vimeo and other video sharing sites, to get more views and to attract a new audiences.

Not Knowing Who Your Audience Is

When you first consider making your first video, it's imperative that you know exactly who your audience is. If you aren't 100% sure who you're talking to, you will not be able to make your topics resonate with them so that you can more viewers. Knowing your audience enables you to know what their goals are, their problems and their success markers, all you have to do them is tailor your content to meet these needs whilst remaining in your industry niche.

Not Keeping Your Topic Narrow

Each video you create should be about a very narrow topic so you can keep them between three and five minutes long, this is the idea length. Once in a while it's okay to go over that, for example if you're teaching someone how to do something step-by-step with screen sharing, but this should be the exception rather than the rule. If you're just talking, the shorter and more to the point your video is, the better as your audience has limited time.

Making Your Videos Too Long

The attention span of your audience is limited and videos that are too long are boring. Even if your topic is interesting, making the video too long often seems boring to your audience. People are in a hurry to get the information they need and don't have time to sit around forever waiting for you to get to the point. If you want people to engage with you, make your videos short and to the point. And don't worry, I struggle with this myself as I have a tendency to want to share more than I should in one video.

Trying to Focus Too Much on Going Viral

As you make your videos you are of course going to think about and try to plan for them going viral, but the simple fact is that you don't know what makes one video go viral and the other not and as such you shouldn't focus on it. You should instead focus on the most important aspect of your video, the message contained within it. You can do all you can to plan for it to go viral by being ready for the onslaught of traffic and more. But, you must still focus on the content instead of the idea it might go viral.

Uploading Only to One Place

The great thing about videos is that, at least for now, you do not have to worry about duplicate content. Posting your video on YouTube, your website, and Vimeo and other video sharing sites is a great idea. The more places you can post it, the better. Enable video editing, and encourage people to share.

Not Promoting Your Video Once Posted

Once you have created a video and posted it, you should promote it. Promote it more than one time, too in fact promote it multiple times, especially if you use Twitter. Make sure you promote it on more than one social media account. Be sure to always comment back when people leave comments for you and try and engage these people in conversations by asking open ended questions. You can promote your video via your blog, social media accounts and more.

If you turn these common video marketing mistakes around, you'll find that your videos become more popular, get more comments, and are shared much more often and your overall content marketing strategy will take a massive step forward.

Content Marketing & Video Production

Content marketing is one of the few forms of marketing that allows you to actively monitor what is and what isn't working, allowing you to make improvements and achieve better and better results. This applies to all forms of content marketing including video marketing and one of the best things you can do every time you put up a video, is to seek feedback from your audience. And believe it or not, the best way to get feedback is simply to ask for it.

From a marketing perspective you want to ask more specific questions, so that you can get the feedback you want. For example, if you got new sound equipment you can ask,

"Let me know if you like how this video sounds."

The more specific you are when asking for feedback from your audience, the better and more useful the feedback will be, let's share a few more tips.

If you adopt a streamlined method of video production by making a similar introduction for each video you post, you'll create a professional impression that will help your audience feel more comfortable leaving feedback.

Make an Exit Video
The exit portion of each video should be similar or the same as well, just like the introduction. This is where you include your call for action, ask for likes, shares, and comments on your video. Being able to easily insert this exit video clip, will help ensure you always ask for feedback.

Embed Other Videos
You can embed links to other videos you have created, even including forms for specialized feedback if you want extra information about what your viewers like or don't like about your videos.

Ask for Likes
You should always ask your audience to like your videos. Sometimes you might want to suggest to them why they should like them instead of just watching them without clicking like. They might not realize

that by clicking like, it actually helps you, to promote your videos and therefore produce more.

Ask for Shares

One of the best types of feedback you'll ever receive is when someone finds your content so good they want to share it with their own audience. All feedback doesn't necessarily have to be a comment; instead think of a share as, "I liked this enough to share it with others and it has a lot of value."

Ask for Ratings

When you want a thumbs up for your video on YouTube for example, you need to ask for it. People are however much more likely to vote something down rather than up. Many people will watch a video without taking any action whatsoever. You should therefore ask for the action you want your audience members to take and more of your audience will do it.

Ask Your Audience for Topic Ideas

A great way to get feedback whilst also increasing audience engagement is to ask your audience for new ideas for topics that you'll cover in future videos. People love having a say in what they watch, so give them a chance to get involved.

Ask Your Audience to Critique the Quality

Sometimes, you want the actual content of the video to be beside the point, but when asking for this type of feedback you have to be specific. Ask your audience how they like the quality, especially if you did something different, purchased new equipment or tried a new technique.

If you really want feedback you're going to have to ask for it, every single time you create and post a video. Your audience will only comment on what they want to, especially if you don't ask for specifics. It also beneficial to try and create something like a video marketing mastermind group, start by giving other video creators feedback, ask for feedback and develop a relationship... in the end you'll all end up helping each other achieve more.

When you first start thinking about incorporating videos into your content marketing mix, one of the best place to get ideas is from your own blog. If you have an active blog and you should, you can use the analytics from Google to figure out which blog posts are the most popular. You can use this information to help you come up with new ideas.

Find out Which Post Are Your Most Popular Blog Posts

Using Google Analytics, determine which blog posts that you have that currently get the most traffic and engagement. These are the topics your audience is telling you they want to know more about.

Rework the Title

You may be able to use the same title, unless you are changing the format. For example, if it's a "top ten" post but you're going to break it up, you'll want to explain that in the title, however you might also like to change the title slightly.

Pick the Most Important Points

Having too many points in a video can make it too long, the idea length of a video is less than five minutes, with some people recommending two to three minutes. So if we take the top ten post mentioned above, instead of taking this list and turning it into a video, why not take one point from each of the top ten posts and turn them into ten separate videos.

Choose Your Technology

Are you going to need a good camera, or will your web cam be good enough? Will you need editing technology to add images, music and other features to your video? Write down what you need so you can determine what you technology is actually required and remember you can often start small and invest over time as your video posts become more popular. A good microphone is one of the smartest investments possible.

Make Slides

If you don't want to make a talking head type video, make slides with one sentence or point per slide that you plan to talk about. You want them to focus on what you're message is, and you should not simply read the slide.

Add Visuals

Images like infographics, memes and graphs work well inside a video. People like to look at more than your head when they see a video. If you use good video editing software, you can add in great images and slides without interrupting the video.

Add Sound Effects

Don't make the music so loud when you're talking that you can't hear what you're saying. However, some royalty free music will make your video look and sound more professional, especially in the intro and exit portion.

Add an Intro and Exit

Prerecord an intro and exit that will be used on all your videos so that you can bring them together into one cohesive valuable asset for your audience, who will learn to instantly recognize your video brand. Don't make them long, though; a few seconds is enough and these can be purchased and used over and over from many well-known outsourcing websites.

Promote Your Videos

Post your video into a new blog post, with a blurb, description, and a transcript. Then also go back to the old blog post and put the link to the video under the old blog post that prompted you to make a video.

Repurposing old blog posts into videos should be your first method of transitioning to adding video to your content marketing mix. Video is more successful than any other form of content in getting more conversions especially these short video bites. But, you don't want to replace everything with video; you just want to add it and reach new audiences and engage everyone better.

Turning your support questions, and forum discussions into videos should be pretty obvious, but to some people it's not. An often undervalued and forgotten area to find video ideas is support questions and discussions in forums or Facebook groups. These areas offer exceptional ideas to spark new video ideas. Don't forget also that we're talking video here but the same applies to blog articles and any content you need for your content marketing.

Look to Your Competition

You don't have to wait for questions to arise in your own discussion groups. Instead, go to the competition's discussion groups and FAQs to find out what questions are being asked. Formulate answers in video form and post to your website, blog, social media and YouTube.

Check LinkedIn

LinkedIn has groups where people start discussions, post articles, and more. Go to the groups that consist of your audience and read the questions they ask. Take any question that relates to your audience and answer it in video form. You can literally find unlimited ideas on LinkedIn.

Read Facebook Groups

Join a few Facebook groups that consist of your audience. When you see people ask questions, don't worry about reading the answers; just collect the questions and use those as ideas for making future videos.

Do a Twitter Search

Look for your niche on Twitter by doing a search on your topic to see if anyone is asking questions about it. Use those questions as your start for any video you want to create.

Check Pinterest

On Pinterest people don't really ask questions, but they do post information in the form of images. They often group things together that they're researching. For example if you have a food blog, and you want to make videos, you can find great recipes for any genre right on Pinterest.

Help Desk Questions

If you have a help desk, whenever you get a question in there, answer it like you normally do but make it in video form. Send the video to the customer, and then post the video in your FAQ for more help when people are searching.

Make a Compilation Video

If you find a lot of the same questions being asked, combine all questions into one subject of the video and try to answer them all in one. Still keep the video short, though.

Ask for Questions

A popular type of longer video on YouTube is a Q & A. Participants ask on social media for questions that they'll answer at a specific date on a future YouTube video. Using this method means you'll have to act fast to answer the questions within 48 to 72 hours of asking your audience to submit their questions.

Using Software to Make Videos

Making videos is easy once you realize that ideas are everywhere. Keep a notepad or Evernote at your fingertips so that you can notate ideas immediately. Don't rely on your memory when you get an idea. Write it down immediately so that you won't miss out on making that video.

When you get stared with video marketing you will quickly realize that you need some sort of software to help you create, edit, and market the videos that you create. It might take a little technical knowledge or the willingness to outsource, but because video marketing is so effective it's important to figure out what you need.

YouTube Editor

A good editor to use for those who don't know how to use the more full-featured editors. You can pull in a lot of clips, put them together, and add transitions and more with this editor.

Link – https://www.youtube.com/editor

Camtasia.com

Full-featured professional level software for video editing. You can record your screen, use it to record your head while talking through a presentation, pull in a video you took with your camera and add transitions, clickable text, and more.

Link – https://www.techsmith.com/camtasia.html

Prezi.com

Making videos from presentation slides is common, but PowerPoint can be really boring these days. You can make even better presentations using Prezi software. Create motion, collaborate with others, use visualization to explain concepts, and personalize the video with your own images, videos and more.

Link – https://prezi.com/

Sellamations

Doodle animation is hot and it's 800 percent more effective than other types of marketing. This is more like a service than software, but it's really important to check it out if you're serious about making money with video marketing.

Link – http://sellamations.com/

GoAnimate

If you want high-end videos with the results to match, try GoAnimate. It has a lot of features that you need to create professional-looking videos with animation. If you want to sell your product or service, this one may help a lot.

Link – http://goanimate.com/

Common Craft

This service plus software enables you to use ready-made videos to explain concepts to your audience, plus the ability to create original videos. It's like PLR for explainer videos.

Link – https://www.commoncraft.com/

EasyVideoSuite

This software puts all the editing features you love into easy-to-use software that even non-techy people can use to create excellent videos. All this at a much lower cost than the professional software, along with easier-to-use features that get results. Made just for people who want to make money online, it works better than other software because it has features you need.

Link – http://easyvideosuite.com/launch/

Speechpad

This really isn't a software product, but it's something that is essential to your success. It's an inexpensive transcription service that will allow you to get exact transcriptions in a variety of different formats to use.

Link – https://www.speechpad.com/

You have to have software for video marketing to be successful. The software that you use will depend on your skill level, budget, and the features that you need. You'll need to figure out what type of videos you want to create; will they be explainer, talking head, animated or a combination of these? As you figure this out, you'll be able to choose the right software for your video marketing needs.

Ways to Maximize Video Marketing

If you want to maximize your video marketing efforts you should look at ways of repurposing the videos that you have created so that you can make the most of your hard work. Using videos in new and engaging ways can help generate more profits and help develop an enormous amount of content.

Put Webinars on Auto Replay

When you present a webinar, record it and put your recorded webinar on auto-play so that people can sign up for the webinar again, and view it as if it was live. Lots of webinar platforms offer this facility and you should take advantage of them.

Cut the Videos to Bite Sized

If you already have videos, you can go through them and find good places to cut them into bite-size short videos that make a specific point of interest to your audience. You can put the videos on social media or as part of a more comprehensive blog post.

Make Shorts into a Longer Video

If you use Vine or Instagram, you can take your visuals that were short and combine them together into one longer video. Add a transcript so that you can get also the most of SEO.

Transcribe Videos

Offer a verbatim transcription of each video as an additional download. Or alternatively post the transcript under the video, it will help search engines find the video and index it accordingly. Some people may prefer to read the transcript to watching the video.

Edit Transcriptions

Take a transcription and alter it to make it more readable and engaging by fixing mistakes, adding images, and making the transcription into a quality piece of content in its own right that you can show on your website or make for sale on its own.

Turn a How to Video into a Blog Post

You may need to cut images out of the video to make the blog post understandable, but making a video into a blog post that stands alone is a great way to make the most of a video.

Curate Your Own Videos

If you have a lot of videos, you can curate them on your website into different categories. This will allow your readers to find your information faster. If you have also transcribed every one of these videos and posted them at the bottom of each video, then your audience will find you faster. Put each video on its own landing page too.

Make eBooks from Webinars

You can take several webinars, transcribe them and put them together to make a very complete eBook. Add some content between the transcriptions, images, and even affiliate links, and you can create an entire information product that starts with an eBook.

Add to a Membership Website

Why don't you make any videos that you've created, along with the other work derived from the videos, into a bundle on a membership website. Memberships are great ways to add income to your bottom line, and adding videos for the members will be very much appreciated.

Podcasts

Often it's possible to take the audio of a video and turn it into a podcast so that people can download and listen to it while they drive to work or whenever they like.

When you repurpose the videos you have created, combine them, transcribe them, and make them into something new, you can really push the boundaries and make the most of the all of the videos you've created. You can increase your audience engagement, revenue and improve your return on investment for each video you create. All it takes is a little forward planning so you make it easy to repurpose later on and boast your video marketing.

There are lots of ways to earn money from the videos that you create, today we're going to look at just one, which just happens to be one of the best which is to create transcripts of the videos and to then repurpose this content in some manner.

Content Centric Advertising

If you use AdSense or some other forms of contextual advertising, which basically means that the advertising service scans the content of your web page and serves the most appropriate advertisement. Posting videos may not be the best way to trigger the right adverts to show up on your website. If you post the transcript directly under the video it will help the search engines pick up the correct search terms and post the most relevant advertisements.

Sell Sponsorships for Posts

You can sell sponsorship packages that you mention during your video and that also are used within the transcript of the video. Charge more for adding their graphic to your transcription of the video, than you charge only to be in the video alone.

Turn the Transcripts into PLR

People are hungry for content, so allow people to use the transcripts of your videos as PLR. This works really well if you're also promoting something that your affiliates are providing. Giving them the permission to use the transcripts as their own can go far in increasing affiliate income.

Make It into a Free Report

If you have some affiliate products which you can add to the transcript such that you can recommend various products or services that relate to the transcript, then you can give something away for free that is monetized within it.

Turn It into a Kindle Series

Transcribe the video and add to it as required, to make it into a small book. If you have a series of videos, this will work very well as you can have a series of books. Give the first away and charge a low fee of about 99 cents to $2.99 for each book in the rest of the series. You can double up on income if you include affiliate links and other offers within the book.

Make YouTube Videos More Searchable

If you have a lot of YouTube videos, you can improve your viewership and make more money if you get them transcribed, upload that transcription to use as closed captioning, and also post the text below the video to help with search engine traffic. Try using Speechpad.com to help accomplish this task.

Convert Transcripts into Articles

For longer videos you can transcribe them, break them up and add extra content to it to make them into individual blog posts or articles. Post these articles alone with still images from the video. You can even post the video again if you want to enable your readers to get more information.

Use Transcripts as Membership Content

Memberships are a great way to earn money, you can add transcripts for all your videos, for premium member content and for those who would rather read than watch a video.

Repurposing videos with transcripts is a great way to earn more money. You can take what you have already done and turn it into multiple different forms that can earn money in its own right and best of all, it helps you maximize your returns as each piece of content works in its own right.

Utilizing tools to make video marketing easier is just darn useful to everyone involved in video marketing. Making videos can be time-consuming, but the payoff is incredible. Video is shared more often than text, and you can turn almost anything you have previously written into a video to share and market to your audience with just a little thought.

Magisto

This is a free video editor that you can use with Chrome. You use it by adding photos and videos and then setting the time drag and dropping your files to create a video with royalty free music to use for your projects. This is only for adding pictures that are turned into a slide show with copy on them.

Link – http://www.magisto.com/

WeVideo

This cloud-based solution allows you to use its powerful tools to edit your videos and make them look really professional. They also have a lot of training available to help you create more professional videos.

Link – https://www.wevideo.com/

Viewbix

If you have three to five minutes, you can create interactive videos out of your videos. Interaction is a great way to help market your products and services as well as make your videos more interesting to watch.

Link – http://corp.viewbix.com/

Camtasia

This is one of the most popular and most often used video editing software. You can produce, edit and upload your videos easily to any network in any format. You can add cool features like clickable links, and you can also add great transitions, voice-overs and more.

Link – https://www.techsmith.com/camtasia.html

YouTube Editor

This tool cannot go unmentioned because it's from YouTube. It's also free. It has some good features, although they are not as advanced as some of the others platforms that you can use. But, you can do a good job with this tool.

Link – https://www.youtube.com/editor

VideoScribe

You've seen the explainer videos, and you've likely seen how expensive they are. This is a little bit of a downgraded version of explainer videos, but it will get the job done while you start out marketing your videos, and for the right price.

Link – http://www.videoscribe.co/buy

Magnet Video

You can create wonderful landing pages, professionally-themed videos, and produce very professional videos to use for marketing your business. This tool even includes content curation tools. You really have to try it to understand all the things this tool does for your video marketing.

Link – http://www.magnetvideo.com/content/marketing+tools/25977

Your Blog

Always post your videos to your blog after you've uploaded them to any video hosting solution. This will make it easier for you to promote the videos to your audience, by making it simple to click a few buttons to share it to social media and your email list.

Social Media Platforms

Remember to promote your videos to all your social media platforms and ask at the end of each video for your viewers to like, follow, share and comment on the videos so that you can get more people to see them.

Choosing to use some of these tools will help make marketing your videos easier, will (after some consistent work) help make your videos engage your audience. Just build momentum over time until you are as successful as you want to be with your video marketing efforts.

Videos in Content Marketing Campaigns

There are lots of ways to use video within your content marketing campaigns, there are lots more than I shall mention here, however these are some great ideas you can use when starting out using video for marketing your business. Let's go over these ideas to help you figure out how you can fit them into your marketing mix.

On Landing Pages

The inclusion of videos on landing pages have been shown to increase conversions by more than 80 percent. It's imperative that a video on a landing page covers enough information to give your viewers the same information that would be on a written sales page. Use trigger words, words on the screen, a talking head, products and more to get your point across.

On LinkedIn

A great way to use a video to help your audience get to know you better is to put an introductory video on LinkedIn. This is a great way to tell people who you are and what you do. Give them a little insight into your world and yourself during the introduction.

In Newsletters

If you send out digital newsletters to your audience, the next level is to attach a video to it. This will encourage your audience to learn more, watch the video, and get excited about your offerings.

On Social Media

Sharing videos on social media is a great way to get more views and to offer your audience something new and often different. Quick, short, to-the-point videos are an awesome way to encourage more engagement.

To Explain a Hard Concept

Video is a great way to explain concepts to your audience that are hard to explain in writing. If you really want to impress your audience, make an explainer video or a demonstration video, to show best what you want to teach your audience.

Demonstrate Your Skills

If you really want to take videos to the next level, use them to show your skills. You can record yourself doing something that you know how to do, speed it up, add some music, and your audience will be in awe.

Show Off Your New Products

When you have new products or services to announce, make a video all about them. It's a better way to explain how things work. And if you are creative enough, it won't matter if it's a product or a service; you can explain it with video.

Let Your Audience In

People love seeing videos about a "day in the life" of the experts they like to watch. If you can let your audience in behind the scenes of what you do, using video, they'll feel even closer to you than before. Thus, their trust will grow, and so will their willingness to buy what you're offering.

Using these ways to market with video will increase your audience engagement and will truly open up a whole new world to you, in the video marketing realm. Video marketing is a highly effective form of online marketing that any business can use and should use.

We've all heard the hype about video marketing being the best and greatest way to improve conversion rates, to engage more and to sell more products however the facts are slightly different. Based on my own research and statistics I have found that the number of people that watch a video is approximately twenty to thirty percent of website visitors and of these up to eighty percent of people are engaged enough to watch to the end. Which is pretty amazing when you consider the bounce rate on most websites, so in my opinion video marketing does work, however it's not the miracle solution most business owners wish it was. However it's impressive enough that everyone should sit up and take notice and add it into their marketing mix, here are a few tips to help.

Business Announcements

A fabulous way to get started with video is to add exciting announcements to your blog using video. Announcements can be made quickly with your webcam and the microphone that comes with your computer and remember people aren't expecting highly professional videos, they want to get to know you.

Customer Testimonials

Ask your customers to make video testimonials or do product reviews for you. It's a great way to add interesting content to your website, social media, and other networks but do please use genuine customers and testimonials as I have seen an influx of video testimonials that in a video classification sense should be rated, fantasy.

Add to Your Email Campaigns

You can actually include videos embedded into your emails with a play button, or include a link to the video inside your email with a description of the video you want your email subscribers to watch.

Show Product Demonstrations

A great use of video is to demonstrate anything to your clients. Whether you have products or services, you can give them examples via video about how to do things such as how to format a blog post on WordPress, or how to bake a cake. It all depends on your niche.

Use in Training

Video is a great thing to use in training for your contractors, affiliates and others. You can teach people how to do simple to complex things via video. It's almost as good as being there in person.

To Show Interviews

Are there movers and shakers in your industry that you'd like to interview? Using Google Hangouts On Air you can gather together a round table of experts, record it, edit it and use it in materials later.

To Cover an Event

Going to a live event? Capture video, put it together, add some annotations, music, and commentary, and you have a wonderful video to share with your audience.

Add Interest to Your Blog with Video Marketing

Text-based blogs can get a little boring. Adding in good pictures, and even a short video within the blog post can add a lot of interest, making it more likely that people will visit, comment and share. You can also add a video introduction to your website instead of the normal blog or home page.

Use on Social Networks

Networks like LinkedIn offer space to put up a video. Why not make a video introduction showing a short compilation of the type of work that you do to viewers who find you there.

Finally, don't forget to remember a call to action with every video. Whether your call to action is to like, share, vote, or buy, it's imperative that you develop a way to leave your viewers with a clear idea of what they should do next, this is what will determine your **video marketing** success after all.

Video Creation of Amazing Attention-Keeping Content

We all want to learn how to create better videos that capture visitors attention and increases conversion rates, the truth is however, that just getting your videos out there is an important step that puts you ahead of your competitors. Contrary to what you might think, you do not have to worry about perfection to use videos for marketing purposes. What you should aim for are well thought out videos, which have been edited to look at least semi-professional and are easy to look at and listen too, get far better results than those that aren't. Here are a few tips to help you to learn how to create better videos.

Plan Your Video

What is the end result of the video that you want to create and who is your audience? If you understand what you're doing going in, it will be easier to keep on task and develop an effective call to action.

Write an Outline

You don't need to write down verbatim what you plan to say, but if you have an outline you can at least check off the topics as you remember to talk about them, it also makes sure you make the points you set out to make.

Get Yourself a Decent Camera

A good camera will enable you to do a lot of clever things, but believe it or not the camera on an iPhone is sufficient… as is your webcam on your laptop if that's all you have. But when you can afford it, get a decent camera to make better videos.

Get Another Recorder

The sound recorder on your camera probably isn't really good enough to record your voice or other sounds as clearly as you'd like. Invest in a decent microphone. Also check the levels on your recording settings.

Check Your Lighting

Perhaps the most important aspects of creating better videos is the lighting. You don't have to spend a ton of money but experiment with different brightness and softness levels and angles of lighting to find what works best for you.

Seek Help

If you want to film other things besides your desk top and yourself speaking directly into the camera, it helps to have a camera person who can hold the camera steady.

Take Lots of Shots

Get many different shots from different angles (awesome tip this), because then you can edit your video down and make it look very good. Even if you only have a camera on your phone, you can still edit it and make it look very professional.

Be Creative

Add in annotations, effects, and clickable links to important facts within your videos, or even link to other related videos. Use sound effects and other effects to make your videos more creative and sharable.

Edit, Edit and Edit

You can use various bits of software to edit your videos to make them better, such as Camtasia Studio, VideoPad, or Movie Maker, or Final Cut Pro if you're a Mac user. Edited and enhanced videos always look better, are shared more often, and get better results.

Links:

Camtasia Studio – http://www.techsmith.com/camtasia.html

VideoPad – http://www.nchsoftware.com/videopad/

Movie Maker – http://windows.microsoft.com/en-us/windows-live/movie-maker#t1=overview

Final Cut Pro – http://www.apple.com/final-cut-pro/

Post Regularly

As with all content marketing, videos that are posted regularly on your website, on YouTube and other areas that are accepting videos and then shared across all your social media sites get the best results. Try to post a video once a week for four months and just look at the results, you might just be amazed.

Learning **how to create better videos** and making your videos stand out from the crowd and get results requires some patience and knowhow. If you're unsure about how to go about doing this, you can always hire a professional even if it's just for the editing. There are many virtual assistants who specialize in this type of multimedia marketing who can help you obtain the results you're looking for.

I often hear people say that video marketing is the future of the Internet, however if you sit and think about it, we're actually following an already established marketing cycle. When people first started to market to one another this was carried out by word of mouth in a similar fashion when the Internet first started it was predominantly based on lots of discussion forums. Then people started to market to each other with print material, then we started to add images, and then we used sound on the radio. When television was invented, we started putting our pictures and text complete with voice-overs on televisions in the form of advertisements.

In the later part of the nineties businesses found the Internet and commercialization began, at this time the Internet was largely text based as bandwidth was limited. Then we started to experiment with audio files and as technology advanced we added more and larger images. Jump forward to today and Internet speeds and upgraded technology such as smart phones and tablets, mean we can watch streaming video from almost anywhere.

So if you think about it, video isn't anything new, but because of the fact that the internet is getting faster and it's getting easier for people to enjoy streaming video, it's just a matter of time before video becomes more important than text based content. Don't get me wrong, text based content will never be replaced but the split between the two will more than likely even out and one will complement the other, especially as one can speed read written content much quicker than watching a video.

Just because we had advertisements on televisions didn't stop us from having advertisements on the radio or within newspapers or magazines. The same will hold true of the Internet, there will always be a variety of different forms of content, as well as different types of advertisements and marketing mediums.

All visual content is going to become more important to go along with your text-based content. Inserting pictures that help illustrate your blog post or article, along with demonstration videos, will go far in making all your content more interesting, engaging, and actionable. Video accomplishes all of that easily. Video is easily to understand, and it's not really that hard to create either, in fact almost anyone can do it.

Visual content like video activates both sides of the viewer's brain, helping them to truly understand and imagine what it would be like to have what they desire and get what they need. There is hardly anything more powerful than the ability to affect both sides of someone's brain when trying to market something to them. They will connect to your brand on an emotional level as well as an intellectual level and this means you will generally sell more.

The advent of more mobile devices with streaming capabilities makes even more likely that video marketing will only become more popular as time rolls forward. Most people, not just children, like to choose to read and view content that has visual elements. If they can have both visual and audio elements, so much the better. That is why the movie industry is so powerful. We love a good story and we love to truly see and visualize how people are affected.

If You Don't Have a Video Marketing Strategy Yet.

It's time to get one, you can start small with very few tools. You just need a camera, or the ability to record your desktop with a software program such as Camtasia Studio, to make a "how to" video for your clients or future customers, and you're in the video marketing game. Just like that. If you don't do it, you're going to be left behind and in business, being left behind means you either spend a lot of time, money and energy catching up or you don't and risk an ever-dwindling order book.

CHAPTER 14: CREATE SOMETHING MAGICAL

Creating Apps

When I started out in the web design business some twenty years back, there were no universities to learn how to do things, we learned on the job in those days and we helped one another learn. Fast forward to today and modern web design is a far cry from designing something that looks good and hoping it will work, today everything is based on proven methodologies and well researched and optimized ways of doing things. We place certain elements onto a page because they work, we know how they work and the results they should generate, in other words nothing is really left to chance, everything is done for a specific purpose and then measured and optimized to generate better than average results.

Today with almost everyone owning a mobile phone, starting a highly in-demand work-at-home business, like app development calls for some very specialized skills. Someone who wants to develop apps needs to know what kind of apps they want to develop, who they want to develop them for, what benefits these people will have using the app and what they need to learn to make it all a reality.

Starting highly in-demand work-at-home businesses, like app development, calls for very specialized skills. Someone who wants to develop apps needs to know what kind of apps they want to develop, who they want to develop them for, and what they need to learn to do it successfully.

If you have the programming skills, start out like you would any business, get a business license, set up a business bank account, set a budget, write a short business plan and get started.

Skills Required for App Development

- Organization

- Leadership

- Creativity and ingenuity

- Market understanding

- Marketing

What's Hot Right Now?
WordPress plugins

Mobile apps

Games

Productivity

Social media apps

Some of the top apps can make upwards of $50K per day, so this is a very lucrative home-based business that you can start with your own ideas. If you have programming skills, you can just get started on your own now. If you don't, that's okay because you can find programmers on sites like Guru.com who will take your idea and create the app for you, while you simply keep coming up with ideas to develop, market and sell.

Getting Started
Come up with an idea for a useful app for your audience, or start developing apps for others for a fee. Either way you decide how you do this business, you can make good money from the comfort of your home. How you set up your business will depend upon whether you want to program apps or come up with the ideas and let other people create the apps. However, the basic steps for getting started are still the same:

- Create a website

- Get a business license

- Create or have an app created

- Market your business

- Give great customer service

- Collect testimonials

- Offer support to your customers

If you want to program apps, figure out who you want to develop them for and market your services to them. If you want to create apps and come up with the ideas on your own it's the same idea in a way. Find your audience, see what they need, create it, and market it directly to them.

Things to Consider

There is no guarantee that your idea will take off and become popular, so be sure to set a budget before getting started.

- Budget – If you hire someone to create an app for you, consider the skill required to do it, and how much you can sell it for. Some apps can be created for as little as $500.

- Fees – If you are a programmer, understand the value of your time and the going rate for creating apps for other business owners in your niche. You don't want to under-price your services or price yourself out of business. Just remember that many a fool has gone out of business being a busy fool and having too much work but not making enough money, I firmly believe everyone in business should charge a suitable and not under-price to gain work.

As you take all the factors into consideration before you start your **app development business**, write down the ideas that you have so that you can create something extraordinary, and remember the secret to business is to manage risks and to never give up.

CHAPTER 15: SELF-CARE

Take Care of Yourself – If You Don't, Who Will?

Taking care of your health and putting time aside to have regular short breaks will also help your productivity and energy levels overall.

With the economic state these days, it's even more important for companies to have reliable employees who are productive and motivated. However, keeping your employees happy shouldn't only be a concern when the economy is suffering. More employers should be considering their employees' wellbeing at all times. Studies have shown employees who are less exposed to stress in the workplace are more productive and healthy.

By considering the following and how they could be implemented into your own business environment, you will show your employees that you are an employer dedicated not only to happiness of your employees, but their overall health as well.

Set clear expectations – By taking the time to ensure every employee is aware of office protocols, you alleviate the potential for any misunderstandings or crossing of boundaries. By doing this you are providing your employees with healthy leadership. Spelling out the office rules and regulations, policies and procedures can be easily accomplished by putting together an office employee manual, as well as taking the time for group and one-on-one discussions.

Make employees feel valued if and when you have them – encourage your employees and offer praise when praise is due. Thank them for a job well done to let them know you value them as part of your team. If a particular situation needs revision, don't approach your employee like a scolding parental figure. Simply review the correct procedure and offer some encouragement. If errors of the same nature continue, you may need to reconsider if this person is in fact a proper fit for the position.

Create a productive atmosphere – The layout of workspaces needs to be considered for maximum productivity. Appropriate working materials and supplies need to be accessible to each employee. They also require enough space to work in an environment which is as comfortable as possible. Ergonomic design could be considered for positive motivation.

Eco-therapy – Another element which assists in a healthy workplace is eco-therapy. Live green plants have an great ability for making the office setting more pleasant, therefore allowing for higher productivity and less stress. The connection to nature while indoors can do wonders for each person's morale. Pictures and murals of nature scenes can also assist in this process.

If possible, allow your employees to keep their office windows open. The benefit of fresh air will keep them healthier. If this is not an option, opt for air-cleaning filters and take responsibility for the maintenance and changing of filters.

Use natural lighting in your office. For workspaces not equipped with window access, install plant light bulbs in all lighting fixtures.

Brain food – Keep healthy snacks available in the office break room. By avoiding junk food, you are giving your employees the opportunity to eat healthier as well as improve moods and positive thinking.

Family time – We all know trying to balance home life and work can be tricky. Make it a policy in your office to allow employees some time off for staying home with sick children, or attending school events without using their vacation time. Consider daycare services either in the same building or at least nearby. Employers who offer daycare services have noticed actual savings resulting from decreased absenteeism.

Healthy work culture – Employers may want to consider holding a seminar for their employees on how to integrate physical fitness into their busy schedules. They can be shown how little chunks of time during the day for stretching or activity breaks can keep them healthy and more productive. Perhaps giving your employees the option to switch their office chair for a pilates ball could help with this as well.

With a little effort and change, not only will your employees be healthier and happier, but your company will win in the end as well. After all, you have the most productive workers in town!

Success Through Being Positive

It's long been accepted that positive thinking can give you a better, happier life, but it can also help boost your business and actually make you more successful.

Successful entrepreneurs need a lot of qualities, but the one that is probably the most important is persistence. Successful businesses often have their failures, but they pick themselves up and keep on going. So what do you do if you're not a naturally persistent person? Change your way of thinking!

If you look at a situation positively, you're going to eventually see the possibilities rather than the failures. That becomes just the push to keep you going, keep you trying and eventually make you more successful.

A positive attitude in general makes you a happier person, and happier people are more appealing to do business with. Sure, people can be annoyed when someone is ALWAYS sunshine and smiles, but they'd much rather deal with someone who is positive and happy than a grumpy person who doesn't see the potential in things.

It's a great idea to start thinking more positively, but if you're like me, it's a lot harder to put into practice. Here are a few steps, some large, some small, that you can take to put a more positive spin on your business and your life.

– Surround yourself with positive people. You can't choose everyone you have to talk to, but you can make sure the people you do choose aren't dragging you down. If you find your husband or a good friend is constantly bringing in negativity, try talking to them and making it a challenge to both turn your thinking around.

– Use positive affirmations. These are positive statements about yourself and your business that you repeat several times at least once a day. Eventually you will find that you start believing these things more and more.

– Make a list of accomplishments. At the end of every day, make a list of what you got done that day, or simply what you've accomplished with your business overall. Make sure nothing is negative and purposely push the negative thoughts from your head. The next day you can read these accomplishments to help give you a positive boost to start your day.

– Take care of yourself. If you feel good, you're more likely to be positive about the world around you. You might find help from exercise and a healthier diet, but can also get benefit from activities like meditation or yoga. They are great for clearing your mind of negative thoughts and giving you a fresh new perspective on life.

If you take small steps to make yourself more positive, you'll probably get some big boosts in your business success.

CHAPTER 16: BUILDING EXPERTISE WITH SELLING & MASTERING THE APPROACH

To really succeed in becoming a millionaire, you need to know how to sell and how to pitch. There's good ways and bad ways to sell. This chapter is going to teach you EXACTLY how to sell – yourself, your business or an item.

How to Create a Unique Selling Proposition that Works

Your unique selling proposition (USP) should explain to your target audience why your company's products and services are preferable to your competitors. Really figuring out and writing down your USP is an important part of developing a profitable business.

To create a good unique selling proposition (USP) you will need to:

Understand Your Target Audience

Who exactly are your target audience, are they married, working, what do they like to do, the more information you can put together the better and most importantly what problems do they have that you can solve?

If you don't know who your target audience is, a quick way to work it out, is to take some of your best clients and work out what they have in common, use this then as the basis for your target audience, and remember the more focused and narrow your target audience the better you are able to connect with them, the larger your audience the harder it becomes which is why saying anyone that can afford my product isn't actually a target market, it's just talk that won't help you engage any audience members.

Get to Know Your Competition

Who is your competition, what are their USP's and how are they serving your audience and what problems do they solve, do they solve them better than you?

Know How Your Product Provides Value

How does your product provide value and solve problems for your audience? Don't get this confused with features of your product, concentrate on value and problem solving.

Know why they should Use You

Why are you the one who should provide the product or service, what makes it really work?

Researching each of the four points above will help you gather the information that you'll need to write your USP. Using the information collected above, you'll want to write your unique selling proposition in a concise, creative way that connects you to your market and explains how you solve their problems and fill their needs differently from your competition, in a way that resonates with your customer.

To write your USP answer the following questions:

- **Product Name** – Write down what you want to name the product.

- **Description of Product** – Describe your product succinctly.

- **How Product Works** – Explain how the product works.

- **How Product Is Different** – Tell your audience how your product is different.

- **Why You Created the Product** – Explain why you created the product or service.

- **Why They Should Buy It** – Tell your audience which problems the product solves.

- **Explain the Guarantee** – This is where you tell them they'll get their money back, or somehow show them that trying your product or service is risk free.

To develop your USP, answering these questions will tell your customers (and anyone involved with your business) what you do, why you do it, and why someone should buy from you. That's what the USP is for, what makes it work is that it's something you and your entire organization can look to when creating new products, services, or for carrying out marketing and sales tasks.

You need to be able to describe the unique benefit to your clients if they purchase your products and services. But, having a clear USP isn't just beneficial to them, it's beneficial for you and your organization too because you need something to focus on, to keep your marketing messages focused and on track.

The other way to make your USP work well is to develop it to be short and concise. After you collect all the information and answer all the questions, you'll use it to write your USP. But once written you will cut out parts and narrow it down immensely. Your entire USP should not be more than a short paragraph of about 50 words or less that you can easily use. Sometimes your USP can become your slogan.

Think of some famous slogans. If they answer who, why, how, what, when, where and make a guarantee, then it's their USP. Think: "The chocolate melts in your mouth, not in your hand."

Of course, you can use your **unique selling proposition** to create an entire story that you can put on your about us page to answer questions your audience has and expand on your short **USP**, that would certainly be much better than most companies about us pages, that drone on about stuff that never engages anyone, let alone your target audience.

How You Approach the Sale with Customers Matters

If you're in business, one of your main activities is making sales, sales leads to profits and without profits you won't have to worry about sales too long as your business will go out of business. Sales is that vital to your business success, and if you accept that it is then it's important to decide on the best ways your business can approach your target audience with offers. Depending on your audience and the product or service that you offer, deciding on the best approach is often the different between closing the sale and losing the sale.

One of the most well-known, as well universally hated sales approaches is the hard sell and we've all been subjected to the hard sell at one time or another. A pushy salesperson that won't take a hint and won't back off is no one's idea of a good purchasing experience. No one wants to be treated like a commodity or an idiot, unfortunately, the hard sell salesperson does both. Why mention it here in this article, simply to warn you never to employ the hard sell approach on your target customers.

If it's not the hard sell then what is the proper approach? Well, the opposite of the hard sell is the soft sell. Now, the soft sell is a legitimate sales approach. In the right hands, through the use of careful suggestion and comments, it can gently persuade a prospective customer to make a purchase. Be careful of the soft sell though, with the wrong product or in the wrongs hands it can fail spectacularly.

A sales approach that has stood the test of time is selling against the competition, which is still widely used because it continues to work. You've probably encountered this approach the last time you went grocery shopping. To sell against the competition, you simply price an item you sell lower than the price your competitors are charging for that same, or similar, item. Customers love to save money and if you can beat your competitor's prices and still remain profitable, then those customers will be beating down your door.

Selling on value is another time honored sales approach and one that I particularly like. When you sell on value you don't stoop to getting into price wars with your competitors, instead, you keep your prices higher and let the customers see the value of your items over the value of your competitor's items. With high-ticket products, this approach is extremely successful. This is because these types of products don't lend themselves to "bargain" sales. After all, who wants cut rate luxury car?

How to Sell to Women

Selling to women is something every online business owner needs to consider, according to the Marketing to Women Conference, eighty-five percent of buying decisions are made by women. This is a massive market segment that you simply cannot ignore or just hope to please, it's therefore an important aspect of online marketing. With more than ninety-four percent of these women having access to the internet, it becomes clearer that you need to appeal to women if you want them to buy, what you have to offer. In fact, some people believe that even if you want a man to buy what you have to offer, you should first appeal to the women in their lives.

Twenty percent of women shop online at least once daily making them the majority of online shoppers. Most women are using mobile devices to access information that helps them make purchasing decisions. With over seventy percent of new businesses being started by women, and many of these being online businesses, it's important for your business to understand the market.

When Selling to Women Make them Feel Special

Women are special, so it's important for you to make them feel that way. Most women report to feeling completely misunderstood by companies. So imagine the advantage your business will have if you make them feel special, this will go beyond the fact that they are women right the way down to your exact particular target audience.

Appeal to Mothers

Most women are mothers or will be mothers or have a mother. If you can appeal to the mother in women, depending upon your audience segment, you can create a powerful urge to purchase your products.

Show that you care about the environment

Women are more environmentally aware today than ever before, if there are two similar products, and one is more environmentally friendly than the other, they'll be more likely to purchase the environmentally friendly model.

Support women's causes

Study your particular audience to find out what causes they care about, then support those causes. Giving ten percent of your profits to a cause that the women in your audience care about will encourage them to buy.

Acknowledge that women love sports

There is a misconception that women do not like sports, but that's just not true. They love sports almost equally to men. Women also like staying fit by walking, running, going to the gym and playing sports.

Be a socially responsible company

Take pride in supporting social causes, because like the environment these are things that a lot of women care about. They want to buy things from companies that share their values.

Create responsive website design

Women use many devices to access the internet so it's important that you design your websites to be responsible, no matter which type of device they use to access your information. Seriously if you're selling to women or men, nowadays your website has to be responsive.

Women are technologically advanced, spending more time online than men, and using more types of devices to access the internet than men.

They tend to buy using whatever device they are using at the time. They buy at their computer, from their mobile devices, as well as in person using their devices to research beforehand.

If **selling to women**, don't misunderstand their intelligence, their autonomy, or their knowledge of social responsibility and the world outside of men. Further, research your audience. If your main criteria for your audience is women, you still have a subset of women that you need to learn about and know.

How to Sell to Men

When selling to men remember that men care a lot about whether or not something works and how it works, they don't really care as much about the story of how the business came to be, or the emotional connections they can make by purchasing the product or service. Men care about how the purchase benefits them, whether or not they can get in and buy the item quickly or not so that they can get back to doing something else.

Selling to Men with Banner and Digital Advertisements.

According to Microsoft, men are more responsive to digital advertisements than women. Even if they don't click through, they see the advertisement on their computer or mobile device and it does influence their choice of whether or not to buy. Men are also more likely to use digital coupons than women.

You Must Be Mobile

Generally, men are using mobile technology to shop while they are at lunch, waiting in line, and doing other activities. The stereotype is mostly true: men don't like to shop. But, they will shop if they need to. If your business website is not responsive, you will lose out on sales because when a man is ready to buy something he's not going to come back later; he's going to buy the item right now, and if not from your website then another website.

Good Search Engine Optimization

Due to the importance of digital advertisements and search engines, having a website that is search engine optimized is imperative. As men usually conduct searches to help them find solutions to problems, if they don't see a banner advertisement, a coupon, or a link on the first page that looks impressive, they're not likely to find you at all.

Social Media and Word of Mouth

While most women value what their significant other says more, men value a combination of factors from what their friends say, as well as what facts the advertisements say. Plus, they care about what is being said on social media. Word of mouth is an important element in helping men choose to make a purchase.

Forget Catalogs

In general, men do not like just looking at catalogs to find what they want to purchase. They like reading quick points about the solution they seek. A few pictures are nice, but they're not going to flip through a catalog to just look at the pictures then find something they want and buy.

Remember, when selling to men, they don't care about the back story as much as women. They want to hear or skim a list of bullet points about a situation and then they want you to fix it, or give them the power to fix it. They like following well-written directions without additional commentary, unlike most women who enjoy the commentary and the back story. Men generally just want the facts and for you to get to the point so remember this when selling to men.

Use the Right Words and You'll Sell More

People love information. If you give them something interesting to read, you can direct them anywhere you choose. Your selling power will experience an increase more than you thought possible.

You are offering quality products or services that you want to sell to the general public to add quality to their lives. The problem is that if the competition is saying the same thing, what will make them choose you?

That is where your wording comes into play. Have you ever read a book and could picture the scene just by the descriptive words on the page? The words made the book come to life.

That is what you will do with the right words. These words will influence the reader to take a look at your website and also to buy or sign up when they get there. These influential words are not just limited to ad copy but can be used throughout your website content and page headlines like a trail of breadcrumbs until they find your product and make the sale.

What are these words? Well, the words vary depending on what you are selling. You want to create a picture with those words of a place or situation that includes your product or service. Once you've created the picture you can begin weaving in words that will have a hypnotic effect on your customers.

To create that picture, you need to know a little something about grammar and sentence structure. As a writer, or if you hire a writer to do the ads, they will need to be familiar with these two things.

Most people read at an eighth-grade level. Big words or long sentences will cause them to yawn and lose interest. Keep your sentences short but powerful. Use as few words as possible to get your point across.

Choosing the right words is like a commercial filled with subliminal messages. It could be a word that appears in several places within the commercial or an action that the actors keep performing that transmits a message to your brain. A sweaty brow could make you feel hot or desire a cold drink or a new air conditioner.

What you don't want is for the customer to figure out what you are doing. It is misdirection as much as persuasion. You are creating a scene that gets the reader to feel certain things while sprinkling in words that will lead them to you and your product. By doing this, when you get to the point where you tell them to visit you and buy, they are ready and eager to do it.

One way to find the right words is to examine other successful businesses and see what they do. What are their "right" words and how do they use them? If you are good at persuasion, choosing the right words for your customer base will bring in the sales you seek.

Millionaires Know They Can Close the Deal

The business world is a cutthroat, dog eat dog environment. Each business is any given field is competing with every other business in that field for a finite amount of customers. Those customers represent sales and the sales convert into profit. If a business isn't profitable, it starves and dies. The choice of words here is intentional, since the similarities between survival in the natural world and in the business world are remarkable.

In both the natural world and the business world, the law of natural selection is at work every day. The entities that are smarter, more efficient, quicker and stronger live to see another day. The entities that make mistakes, are afraid to take initiative, forget to protect their backs and simply can't run fast enough become the fuel for the entities who do survive. If this sounds ruthless, it is. To survive you have to want to survive. More so, you have to believe that you can survive.

If you fail to have enough confidence to believe in yourself, you will never survive in the business world. It's that simple. In addition, if you have no faith or confidence in the products or services you are selling you will also fail. You need self-confidence, as well as a belief that what you sell is the best available in order to succeed.

People, like your customers, can sense confidence. As human beings, we have evolved to understand a myriad of non-verbal cues that operate on our psyches on a subconscious level. We used these cues in the past to survive. They helped us to determine who was a friend or who was an enemy. They are still operating on us today. Only know instead of helping us determine ally or foe, they help us determine who to trust and who not to trust.

When you believe in yourself and in what you do, people see it without you having to say a word. This self-belief then helps them to judge you positively as a person that they can trust. This trust, in turn, then becomes the basis for building a bridge of confidence that leads, in the end, to a sale.

Every successful salesperson understands this subconscious form of communication. They also understand that if they fail to believe in themselves, their potential customers will sense this and interpret the information as a reason not to develop trust. The end result is lost sales.

Expand the Lifetime Value of Your Client/Customer

As a business owner you most likely know that each customer has a lifetime value to your business. This is often called the CLV or customer lifetime value. It roughly translates into the amount that you can earn from any one customer as they enter your product funnel. For example we all purchase food, so if you're like me and tend to shop in the same shops week after week, year after year then the total amount of money I spend during these years of continuous shopping represents to the business my lifetime value. Understanding your CLV can help determine ways to expand your CLV.

Be More Customer Centric

Customer service is one of the most important parts of any business. Even if you have the best products or services in the world, if your customer service is lacking you won't last long as your customers won't like you. If you want repeat buyers, treat your customers with the importance and respect they deserve.

Build Targeted Upsells

With technology like LeadPages.net you can easily create an automated system to build up-selling opportunities into your customers buying process. For example, you might like to do it in the shopping cart itself, or you can do it through follow-up emails.

Create Logical Cross-Sells

A cross-sell is a just selling a different product to a current customer. It should relate to your audience, but it doesn't have to relate to the other product that you sold them the same way an upsell generally does.

Be Responsive

It's imperative that you set up a system that makes you seem super responsive to your customers. Whether that's an automated ticketing system, a 48-hour answering policy, or open office hours doesn't matter. But, you need to be perceived as being very responsive to keep your customers happy.

Over Deliver

Every product or service that you deliver should be better than the customer expects. The fact is, you won't please everyone all the time, but you can always aim to over deliver. If a customer is unhappy, you can over deliver with your solution to fix their problem thus turning problems into future opportunities.

Create a Referral Program

Let your customers earn money or discount points by recommending you to other people. Often, when people can earn enough money to support their buying habits, they'll be more likely to spend money with you. It's a win-win all the way around.

Stay Connected

Find ways to stay connected with your audience, such as social media, email, teleseminars, and webinars. The more ways they can connect with you, the happier they're going to be and the more your CLV will expand.

Develop an Inner Circle

One way to expand your CLV is to provide a fee-based inner circle that certain customers can join. It can be on a private forum or even utilize a private Facebook group or create your own forum with native software.

Nothing is more important in your business than your customers, understand and accept this so that it is at the core of everything you do. The more you can study what your customers need and find a way to deliver it to them, the longer they'll stick with you. But, you have to keep creating products to keep those who've bought from you interested and wanting more.

CHAPTER 17: PRODUCT & RETAIL MANAGEMENT

Cross-Selling & Upselling

Cross selling and upselling are both great ways to add additional revenue to your bottom line, both attempt to encourage the customer to purchase additional products and spend more money.

When cross selling a customer will adds in more products from a complementary category that may or may not be related to the same category as the original item purchased, and purchasers aren't required to make the other purchase to get it. Let me give you an example, you sell book called "how to perfect your golf swing" you could then recommend other products, or cross sell items such as golf gloves, golf balls, golf training aids, clothes, etc. All are related in some way to the original product but you cross categories from books to other products.

Now let's look at upselling, an upsell adds more products from the same category. Let's look at our example above of selling a book about perfecting your golf swing. You could then upsell a book plus a DVD package of the book that shows examples of the lessons contained within the book. You could also add on a membership to a group training sessions, perhaps then one on one golf lessons. All of these are an on add on to the book to help the purchaser use the book properly, you have to buy the book to get the other products.

All of this is value added selling, McDonald's and their "would you like fries with that?" question is perhaps the most famous value add of all times and has generated millions, perhaps billions of dollars. Sales people do these forms of selling every day to increase their bottom lines, the secret is to find ways that you can do it also.

Upselling Ideas

Upselling requires some product planning in order to work. You'll need to offer your product in a few different forms so that when customers click on one product they'll automatically be recommended to buy the better upgraded package of the same product with more benefits for them.

One of the best ways to upsell items is to do it directly within the shopping cart, if possible after a user has made the decision to make a purchase and has added the item to a shopping cart. Simply offer more choices within the cart to add on to the purchase they are already making. If you cannot do it this way, send them to a thank you page after they have made their purchase that offers the additional items to add to their package to get the upgraded super-sized version of the product.

Cross Selling Ideas

Cross selling on the other hand is simply a natural progression on to the item they are purchasing. If you are selling eBooks, natural items you could cross sell are eBook readers, reading lights, eBook cases, and anything related to eBooks for that matter.

What's more, if you sell eBooks about specific topics, you can cross-sell items related to those topics. For instance if you sell golf books you can then also sell golf training aids, golf equipment, golf clothing and much, much more.

As long as what you're cross selling is somehow relevant to the purchaser, you can recommend it. Many shopping carts, website product listings, etc… now allow you to show related products to the item being purchased. You also see on some of the better shopping carts, a facility that shows customers a list of items other customers purchased when they bought the item they have just bought. The potential to earn more money through cross selling are tremendous.

Upselling and cross selling need to become part of your entire sales funnel, if you don't offer upselling and cross selling opportunities, just ask yourself how many dollars you are leaving on the table.

CHAPTER 18: BRANDING

Branded Websites

Every single business needs to have a perfectly branded website, as this is the place where all of your online marketing efforts begin and end, it's the center of your universe and all of your social media and other online marketing channels act as satellites directing people back to your website.

Having just any old website will not do your business any favors, in fact it's more than likely to do the opposite and help drive potential customers away. To help ensure you have a perfectly branded website, follow these few steps.

Choose Your Domain Name Wisely

If you already have a name for your business, your domain name should typically match it. If you cannot purchase the exact name, because someone else has it, consider using keywords or keyword phrases that match what you do in your business instead. Be careful here, though. If you change your products or services later, you may have to start over.

Use a Reliable Hosting Service

While this may not seem to be related to your brand, it is because you want your hosting company to be very reliable so that your website does not have much, if any down time because most people will not revisit a website they find that is offline. If they click through on some of your advertising and end up on an error page due to the fact that your website has crashed or is down, they probably won't come back. It's also worth checking out what support your hosting company offers and how easy it is to contact them when something goes wrong.

Design User-Friendly Navigation

No one likes going to a website and being unable to find what they are looking for, so try to make it super easy for your visitors to find everything on your website by having multiples types of website navigation and multiple ways to contact you. Don't try to have a flash navigation system that no one understands, have your home button top left and contact us far right, why? Because this is where people expect to find them and by doing this you'll give people what they expect and you'll get more click-throughs.

Create an Attractive Layout

The layout of your website should be pleasing to the eye, match your other marketing materials and evoke the emotions you want it to, based on your brand's image. It should be responsive and work on multiple devices, oh and if your website is not responsive you are losing out big-time as more people now access the Internet via mobile devices than by computer and these people are not going to your website unless its responsive.

Blog Regularly and with a Purpose

It's not enough to just have a blog that you update every now and again. You need a blog that has targeted information relating to your business written for your targeted audience. The blog posts should be smart, unique, and speak to your audience as well as use keywords that attract search engine traffic and you must update your blog regularly and to a schedule your audience can learn and therefore can anticipate new content.

Keep All Information Updated

Aside from a blog that is updated on a regular basis, it is important that other information on your website is also kept updated. If you've listed your staff on your website, and someone leaves or someone else joins make it a priority to update this information. This applies to all information as people don't want to read about past events, outdated news or anything that isn't currently applicable, so keep it updated and your audience engaged.

It's also important to always keep promoting your website via your social media accounts and every other means you know about and understand The more you promote your website, the more likely you are to want to keep it current and relevant to your audience. You should be proud of your website, and it should form one of the key ingredients of your marketing plan.

Any type of marketing done online should be aimed at directing people back to your website – whether it's to go to the website to fill out a form, to read a blog post, to watch a video, to sign up for a contest, or to buy something. The website is the center of your online universe and everything else satellites directing people back.

CHAPTER 19: SHARING

The Heart of Social Media

Sharing is at the heart of social media. It's how participants start a conversation about something. They share it. But first, your content has to be worth sharing. It has to provoke enough thought about it for someone to like it, Google+ it and share it on other social media formats. But, how do you make sure you create content that is share-worthy?

Share Everything Yourself

First, get in the habit of sharing things yourself. Share your blog posts, your YouTube videos and any content that you create on your social media. How often you share something depends on which social media you are using. Remember that people are sitting in wait for your shares and they don't typically scroll back to find out if they missed anything. Therefore it's up to you to find out the best time of day to share, and how often to share, based on which social media you're using.

Ask People to Share

Always remember to include a call to action within your content. You want to tell people to "like" you, "share" and "g+" you. They truly may not think of doing it without your directions. It's not that they don't like your content it's just that most people are oblivious to the power of sharing and so they just don't do it. Include the asking in your call to action every single time and you'll get more shares right away.

Keep Your Social Shares Short

Twitter forces brevity, but Facebook doesn't. However, studies show that shorter posts on Facebook get more shares than longer ones. So, use the ability to put a link to the main source of content in your shares and make your comments short on the actual social media. Make the comment get noticed by asking a question or asking for action with a headline that will get attention from your followers.

Pay Attention to What Your Share Looks Like

What does the viewer see when they see your share? Do they see an image that gets their attention? Do they see words that make them want to read more? What exactly do they see on their end? It's important to understand how size of images, and the automatic cropping of them on social media plays into whether someone wants to view or share your information or not.

Finally, be sure that you've done adequate research on your target audience so that you know what they want. If you are not sharing the type of information your target audience wants, then you may end up with a lot of shares and likes from people who are the wrong audience. Keep your audience in mind for everything you do and you'll be more successful in getting more shares with your social media.

CHAPTER 20: DIVERSIFICATION IN SERVICE/PRODUCT OFFERINGS

Create Membership Sites that are Unique and Original

Many people are creating membership sites to make extra money, and they're doing it because it works. Membership sites are one of the best ways to make money on the internet. Think about it – even companies like Amazon.com are offering a membership to get your items shipped faster and enable you to view unlimited videos. If membership didn't work, they would not try it.

1. It's the Best Way to Make Money Online

Membership sites are literally one of the most lucrative ways to make money online. Some people are earning more than six figures with their membership site websites each year. Once you've created the site, especially if you create a limited time membership, your work is done. Other than the marketing part, and guess what – you can pay members to market it for you, making this as hands off as possible. It's as easy as "set it and forget it" in terms of ways to make money on the net. Plus with the technology available today, it's easy to get started.

2. They're Easy to Set Up and Run

Due to the technology available today, almost anyone can run some form of a membership site – whether it's a limited time membership site, an email membership ecourse, or a full-fledged membership site with a forum and often updated content. It's up to you which type you use. But, the technology exists to create any and all of the above rather easily and inexpensively. What's more, you can easily outsource most of it if you have the budget.

3. Membership Sites Are Great Entry Points for Affiliates

Good affiliates like to try out products before they promote them. Many types of membership software has the ability to offer members only an affiliate link to promote the membership as well as other products that you develop. Since the new affiliate gets to see what your products are like via the membership site, they'll be more likely to want to promote what you are offering.

4. They're Awesome Ways to Connect Directly with Your Audience

You're a busy person, so it can be difficult to find the time to connect on an individual basis with your audience. But, with a membership site you can reach a lot of people without as much effort. You can create weekly podcasts, or video casts, or even have monthly webinars and/or teleseminars just for members. They'll feel special; you'll connect with many of them in a way that feels good to them, and maybe even convert some of them to more direct and more expensive inner circle connections if that's what you want to do.

5. It's Almost Passive Income

Recurring revenue is the carrot that draws business owners to building membership websites, and recurring revenue is what keeps them doing it, year after year. Many membership tycoons create niche membership site after niche membership site, repeating their success over and over. Due to the technology that exists today, it's practically passive income once you have it set up. What more reasons do you need to get started creating your membership site today?

There are so many different types of membership site that you're sure to find the one that works for you. You can do it as hands off as you want, or as hands on as you want. It's totally up to you, the technology you choose, and your niche.

I know of people that are making a great living by running a membership website and I believe that with the right plan you can make a full time living only by adding membership to your product range. Personally I love the residual income that membership websites offer and it also helps maximize revenue streams.

Here are ten reasons why membership is lucrative:

1. You'll Feel Good

When you can offer something to others that they need and want, you're going to feel positive about it. This makes a membership website more lucrative because you're going to not only make money, but you are also going to want to keep adding to it, giving more and more value. Which in turn means that going to work actually becomes fun, and you end up going having fun all day.

2. Low Initial Costs to Start a Membership Website

Provided you choose your software properly and take into consideration your own level of knowledge, the start-up costs are reasonably low, and well within the reach of most people.

3. Residual Income

If you haven't experienced the joy of residual income which means the consistency of a regular income, you will when you start a successful membership website. People start them for a reason, and people also join them for the same reason.

4. People Like Privacy

Members join a club for privacy because they can go to a membership site and talk about what they want to without worry that it's searchable by clients and associates on the internet.

5. You Can Do It Alone

You don't need a huge staff to help you build or run a successful membership website, in fact I know of one that boasts of over a thousand members that is run by one person. Once you get the technology set up, you just have to add to it on a regular basis and participate in discussions in the forums. If you do a drip membership, you can set it up and forget it, less staff equals more profit and a drip membership means that you stagger the content that you have to new members, so that each month something else is automatically dripped to them, without you having to add anything, although you should ensure it is updated from time to time.

6. You Have Something to Offer

Anyone who has something to offer, that others perceive of value, even if it's the smallest niche can start a membership website that is successful.

7. Add Value to Your Current Business

If you already have a business presence online, adding a membership program will often take your business to the next level, remember it's the perception of your audience that counts.

8. People Want Exclusivity

Membership makes people feel special, elite if you like, as if they're part of a secret group of movers and shakers. Therefore, getting people to join isn't hard as human nature drives them to get involved. Getting them to remain members is a little more work but if you focus on value, value and more value, you will do it.

9. People Expect a ROI

People join membership sites expecting to get massive value out of the membership. And as long as you can provide that to them, then not only will they feel they're getting a return on their investment, you will too as they will hang about.

10. People Are Curious

People will join simply out of curiosity to see what's inside. It's up to you to hold them there to increase your profits, and if you have lots of initial value and are using a drip type membership you could consider offering a free trial membership.

If you market your membership website correctly, you will have a successful online membership business, provided that you've done your homework on starting it in the right niche and provided you give real value. People want to feel as if they belong and are part of a community, and they like having privacy. If you have information to offer, **a membership website is a great way to do it** and remember all of those members are out there often acting as great sources of referrals.

Have you noticed that many businesses utilize a membership business model and most of us don't even realize, we're so comfortable with it? For example I can remember joining a video club and showing my membership card every time I wanted to rent something, I've been a member of a gym, a drinking establishment and even a golf club. It's obvious the concept is lucrative but how do memberships, really generate income and why?

People Love Feeling As If They Belong

Being part of a community of like mined people who have the same interests as you do is very powerful. They say birds of a feather flock together, and memberships prove this point over and over again. Your business can have a very small niche and still attract members in enough numbers to be profitable if you price the membership right and deliver ongoing value.

You Offer Unique High Value Products

No online membership is complete without something new, at least on a monthly basis be it a new products or services added to keep the members interested. The products need to add value to the consumer to the point that they say, "Wow, this is awesome."

Participate in the Forum Personally

Discussion forums are the lifeblood of any membership website, they allow members to interact with each other and form relationships. Without a discussion forum you will have very little opportunity to keep your audience excited and willing to pay the membership fee month after month. You should spend time on the forum every single day, so that you deliver value and build lasting relationships.

Your Content Is Regularly Updated

Aside from products and services, the content that your members consume each month is important too. You need to update content daily (if possible) with a blog post, plus contribute more content each month such as white papers, checklists and so forth, so that you are constantly adding in value.

You Know How to Over Deliver

It's all too easy get carried away with marketing and make your audience feel as if they're going to get more than they actually are. This is always a mistake, membership websites that make money deliver far more value than the person joining believes they'll get.

Start-up Costs Are Relatively Low

All you need to start a site is a way to make sales pages, landing pages, a membership website complete with membership, plus an email auto-responder and discussion forum. You can install it all yourself or hire someone, and be up and running for a relatively small cost with some form of ongoing expenses, depending on the software and platform you select.

You Can Charge More People Less for Superior Value

Another major attraction people have to memberships is that it is a way to spread the cost of resources over many different people. Something that might cost thousands a month for one-on-one work will now cost just a fraction of that when you spread that cost over many different members.

Offer Unannounced Extras

Another neat trick to keep members interested in your offering is to offer unannounced extras that make your members want to see what comes each month. Make these really special and super hyper-focused on the audience, and you'll have a winning combination, that will ensure members remain members for a long time.

Earning money from membership sites is easier than many other methods of earning money online, but you do have to continuously wow your audience to keep them interested, plus devote a fair amount of time to marketing the membership itself. Always remember to try and drip feed content to new members and to recognize long time members within your community.

Creating a membership website is a lot of fun, but it's often hard to think of what to include within it. The vast majority of websites offer their members similar offerings and although you need to at least stick to these basics. I would advise you to go beyond that, because the more you can pack into your membership area, the more in demand your membership will become and the better your membership retention will be.

Glossary

This could be a list of resources as well as a list of terms so that members can easily understand all of the terms used in the content, information products, videos, forum, etc. It's always best to assume that some of your audience don't understand everything, a glossary allows you to explain everything that you can.

Message Board

The most popular membership websites have a forum or message board for members to speak to each other as well as to the leaders and coaches who are running the membership site. It builds community, and I know of people remaining members of membership website simply to continue the regular engagement with their friends on these forums.

Permanent and Temporary Content

Ideally your membership website wants both temporary and more permanent content to continuously flow through the site. The core content of the membership site should be around all the time and some should drip in based on where a member is in their membership program. This will help you retain members as something new is always coming and it's this knowledge and fear of missing out that keeps people hanging around.

Videos

Utilizing video is always a good thing in a membership website, in fact this is the most often used resource for passing information over to members. Whether it's a "how to" do something, interviews, courses, or something else, video always enhances a membership website. You can use PowerPoint and your own voice to produce videos easily, and this is how I do most of the ones I use.

eCourses

Learning how to do something is a good reason to join a membership site and if you have a few courses that your members can get a certificate for finishing, all the better. It will make them want to stick around and complete the course. Once again with modern technology this isn't that hard to implement.

Information Products

At least once a month, include a full-fledged new information product for the membership to use and implement. Information products can include eBooks, video, eCourses, and more but can also be sold individually on their own outside of the membership, allowing you to maximize revenue.

Checklists

If you are like me, then you love a good checklist that you can follow along with to get things done. You can include checklists about how to use the membership website as well as checklists about how to do something your audience wants to do. There are so many options for you to fill your membership up with, that will prove useful to your members.

You

The most important resource to include in your membership site is you. You must be actively involved within the forum, with making videos, with writing content and as a cheerleader for your members, especially cheerleading. That's why people are joining, after all.

Filling your membership site up with useful and unique resources should become your long term goal and something you are passionate about especially as your members grow. You'll get lots of ideas directly from the members, so don't worry just ask them in the forums. The important thing is to get started with a minimum and build as you go along to make your membership more valuable with each passing month.

When you start any new business you should always write a business plan. A business plan will help you determine what type of technology you need, what niche you want to target, what products and services you'll offer your membership and exactly how you plan to deliver it and market it. Without a business plan, you're just shooting in the dark and you're probably going to miss.

Your business plan can be just one page and should include:

1. Describe the audience you want to reach – Write a sentence or two that describes your audience. Perhaps create a persona of the person you want to reach so that you know who to direct all your marketing material toward.

2. Describe the problems your membership solves – What problems will you solve for your target audience? Be very clear; in one or two sentences write out what problems you solve for the persona you created above.

3. List your top two or three competitors – It's important that you look into who you're competing with. Find them, and list them. Explain why they're competitors and why you're different/better.

4. List the products, services and price points you will offer – This is really your product funnel. If you can draw a picture of your product funnel and how you'll pull people into your funnel, describe how you will eventually get them to join your membership, what you plan to charge, and what will keep them there, you've got it made.

5. Describe how you will market your membership site – Use the information above to describe exactly how you will market your membership site. List your marketing budget in dollars.

6. Describe who will create products and provide services – If it's all you, say so, and describe your qualifications. If you will outsource, describe who and in both cases write down the cost of creating products and performing services.

7. List your expenses – Outside of product creation you'll need to list all your expenses. Don't forget rent, technology, online and offline expenses that you will have every month in your business.

8. Get real with the numbers – Describe exactly what constitutes success with your membership site. How many members do you need to break even; how many members do you need to make a profit?

9. Put your plan in writing – Finalize your plan and put it in writing. This will give you an easy document to look at as you're moving forward with your membership site development, marketing, and servicing.

Even a one-page business plan can help you make a success of your membership site. Don't just jump into any new business idea without studying all the factors that go into a business plan. It doesn't mean you have to write it in a 20-page report. You can write it down on only one page and be successful.

Membership sites are an excellent way to increase revenue and develop a recurring revenue stream. What makes membership sites so easy to run and virtual money-making machines is the technology that runs it all. The membership site software you choose will depend on your skill level and whether you're going to hire a technology expert to work with you or not.

Here are a few software options for all skill levels.

* EasyMemberPro.com – This is powerful and easy-to-use membership software that runs on your web hosting service. It is made to be user friendly and integrates with many autoresponders, WordPress, and forums. It has a built-in affiliate program manager, automatic backups so you don't have to worry, coupon codes, one-time offers, up-sells, unlimited site licenses, easy member management and more.

* AMember.com – One of the favorites of membership site creators, aMember Pro has many features such as free installation, an affiliate module and integrated helpdesk, and it works with WordPress sites too. You can have unlimited membership levels as well as drip content delivery and even email management if you choose to use it. It's a one-time fee unless you want to upgrade, and it is installed on your server.

* Kajabi.com – This membership site software is cloud based and carries a monthly fee. The good thing about that is you don't have to deal with the technology end of things as much as you might with self-hosted membership software. Kajabi has many features such as automatic content delivery, easy to create squeeze pages, landing pages, drip technology, commenting and discussion forums, and more. You can try it out free.

* MemberPress.com – This is a WordPress plug-in that will help you create awesome membership sites with your current WordPress site. You can control content access, sell digital products, accept payments right on your site, and build really good membership sites. It integrates with AWeber and MailChimp. It also integrates with WordPress-based forums like bbPress and Simple Press Forum if you should care to have a discussion forum with your membership site.

* SiteManPro.com – This software works with WordPress by using MemberPlug and even static HTML websites. You can build a membership site that is very powerful with this software and you can also manage them all from one dashboard. This software has everything from license management to integrations with other products like Zendesk.com (which is hosted helpdesk software). You have a choice of a yearly fee or even a lifetime purchase of this software. What's more, they even install it on your server, for free.

Membership sites are big business and so is the technology behind building a successful membership website. Choose carefully. If you are a member of a site now that you enjoy using, why not inquire as to which software they use. Typically, people are happy to share what membership site software they use, especially if they happen to be affiliates of the software and can make a small profit from your purchase.

When you start making money on the internet, you want to find a way to earn a recurring income. Most people start out with a few information products, work their way up to coaching, and eventually realize that the best way to earn recurring revenue is via membership sites.

A membership site doesn't have to be complicated. There is a lot of technology out there to help you create a very well made membership site. When you think about how much money you want to make on the internet, it becomes quickly apparent that making money with membership sites is the way to go.

Let's say you want to make an additional $3000 per month. You have a lot of information products, you're a known expert in your niche, maybe you even have a popular and expensive one-on-one coaching business. If you're willing to invest in the technology required, and the help to monitor the membership, you can very easily do this.

If you only charged $30.00 per member per month, which is actually a low price if you're that big of an expert, you only need 100 members to bring in that additional $3000 dollars a month, each and every month. 100 members is a drop in the bucket when you consider the numbers of people who are interested in your niche.

If you don't want to go that big, there are other ways to create membership sites that are profitable. You can create an eCourse that is 12 weeks long, charge a fee each week to keep getting the information delivered by email and you have yourself a membership site without even having the website membership technology in place. All you need to do is use something like AWeber and PayPal to get started.

To have a profitable membership site you need:

A Niche You're Passionate About

You likely already have a niche but if you don't, do your homework to find a money-making niche where you will have no problems coming up with at least one good product each month, or week, depending on what you're planning to promise the membership. What's really great is you can actually create your first product, then create the products on schedule after you're already attracting members. No need to create 52 products before you start marketing.

Information to Disseminate to the Members

Start with at least some information that you can provide the members when they join. Often membership sites that are on a website have access to a discussion board where members can speak to and among each other about the products and services the membership provides. Then there is a members' area where members can download the information they get with their membership each period that you've decided upon. As mentioned above, you can start with just one period of information and add to it as you market the membership.

Membership Site Technology

There are a lot of different styles of membership sites, and a lot of different software and technology to make it happen. The features you want to offer your members will help you make the choice of what type of membership technology you want to implement.

You don't have to have a message board if you don't want one. You can deliver all membership material via email if you prefer, or you can create a website with the downloadable products available by links that are sent via email autoresponder software on a periodic basis. Make a list of the features you want, then look for the software.

Loyal Fans and Followers Who Want the Information You Have

Your membership site will be more fruitful if you already have a loyal following and this is a new offer in your product funnel. If you already have books, reports, services, information, coaching, and more, you're primed for starting a membership site and making it super profitable. But, even if you don't have that many fans or followers yet, you can build them with the right niche.

Getting started is the key to making money with membership sites. Don't let the idea overwhelm you; membership sites are a great addition to your product funnel if you really want to create long-term recurring revenue in your business.

Creating a profitable membership site is the dream of many online entrepreneurs. It's no wonder, because the profits can be huge with the right membership site created for just the right market and the right niche. When you consider that a membership site that only charges $10 dollars a month can bring in an additional 1000 dollars of profit each month with just 100 members, you can quickly start realizing the power of a well-created, profitable membership site.

Know Your Market

Maybe you get tired of reading it, but you must know your market. Research your market to find out what they want in a membership site and whether or not such a thing would interest them. You can send a survey to your existing market to find out their interest in a membership opportunity and even what price point would best suit them. Based on that information you can create just the right membership site opportunity.

Understand Your Product Funnel

Your product funnel probably looks something like this: you offer a small report or other inexpensive (or even free item) to your target audience to get them on your email list. You then market your more expensive information products, they purchase something a little more expensive, and then you move them down your product funnel until they've bought the most expensive item you have – which might be one-on-one coaching or an email course.

Then they're gone. In fact, most probably don't even buy your one-on-one coaching because it's so expensive (and rightly so). To add in a membership opportunity to your list, simply start marketing the opportunity before your one-on-one coaching as a way for people to get more connected with you. You'll likely sell more one-on-one coaching to members than you will to anyone else, which will make your membership site even more profitable.

Offer Exclusive Products and Services

Aside from your regular offerings that you provide to anyone, your membership site needs to offer products and services that no one else can get unless they are a member. By making members feel exclusive, you'll encourage them to join and to stick around. To keep creating good products, remember to stay very focused on your niche and don't move outside of that niche for your membership site. You don't want to confuse your members.

Under Promise and Over Deliver

Another component of a profitable membership site is to practice under promising and over delivering. You do want to brag about your awesome membership site and all that it provides to members, of course, but you want to throw in some extras that only the members know about. This will encourage them to stick around, creating the recurring revenue that you need to make membership sites profitable.

Create Scarcity with Limited Memberships

If you're priced your membership well, you might consider limiting the number of members that can be involved. This works especially well if you plan to spend a considerable amount of your time coaching members via message board, webinars, or other specials that you provide to members.

Limiting to even fifty members can create a situation where you literally have a waiting list to get in. Even if you charged 100 dollars a month, which is not unreasonable when you're only allowing fifty members in, that's an additional 5000 dollars a month. Tip: If this works well, and you feel like you have more time, create an additional copy of the membership model with a slightly different focus but which can use some of the same materials.

Find Well-Working Automated Technology

One of the biggest components in creating a profitable membership site is to find the right technology that delivers what you need. Some membership site software can deliver "drip" content so that members do not receive all that you offer the first day they sign on. Yet others offer several levels of exclusivity to members with the ability to offer an inexpensive membership and move up levels for access to the most expensive and most exclusive offering. To really be effective the technology must be automated so members don't get frustrated and you don't have to work yourself to death.

You may decide that a membership site is something you want to do, and if that is the case, consider your expertise, narrow down your niche, and get started on creating your profitable membership site as soon as possible. You can get help creating your membership site by hiring people who are experts in membership site technology and understand the components that make membership sites profitable.

Going Audio

When using audio online to market your business, it's important to keep abreast of current trends to try and predict what will happen in the future and by listening to your audience you can find out what's important today. When predicting the future you have to remember that some things may become true whilst others will not, and some things you haven't thought about might push to the forefront. But, if you're prepared for change, you can often make it as needed to accommodate new trends and to be seen as someone with a finger on the pulse, to help here are some trends to watch for in 2015.

Providing More and More Value Will Become More Important

Consumers are almost demanding more and more value for their dollar, as always. But, when it comes to audio they're becoming accustomed to high quality productions. The good news is the technology to produce high quality audio and provide value to your audience isn't expensive. With the most expensive thing you would typically purchase being a good microphone.

Customer Centric Audio Products Will Increase

More and more consumers will want to listen to audio products rather than reading print products. People can listen to audio while doing other activities and most people enjoy doing more than one thing at a time these days, such as driving and listening which I must admit I love to do.

Online Communities will Increase as Will Their Importance

With the advent of Facebook groups, smart business owners are harnessing the power of online communities. Starting forums and private membership sites in which to distribute your audio to your audience is an excellent way for a business owners to use this avenue.

Acknowledging Mobile Influence on Audio

There is no doubt that mobile is a huge game changer for everyone who has an online business or wants to market their business online, it's not happening it's already happened. Now mobile cannot be an afterthought, it has to be part of your master plan.

Podcasting Will Become More Prevalent

Due to the fact that technology is getting less and less expensive and the barriers to entry have lessened to almost nothing, more business owners will engage in podcasting as a way to distribute information to their audiences.

Provide Paid and Free Content that Work Well Together

As the future comes upon us, smart business owners will need to find ways to incorporate both paid and free content for their audiences to digest. For example, you might have a few free podcasts on your website for your visitors to listen to, but then direct them to iTunes to find and purchase more.

Original Audio Content Will Set the Standard

As the audience gets used to fresh original content, the demand will become even greater for more and more content. The audience is truly insatiable, which is why you have to always be on the lookout for ways to create more original content.

Audio Quality Will Become More Important as Competition Increases

As more business owners enter the audio marketing channel, your audio products need to increase in quality in order to compete. Invest in the right tools, and try to produce professional results. As a minimum I would suggest having an introduction and closing sequence professionally produced, with your audio sitting in between.

Teleseminars Will Continue Being Popular

Even with the popularity of webinars, teleseminars are still popular and will continue to be popular ways to get a lot of information out to lots of people at one time.

Watch out for these trends in 2015 with regard to using audio marketing in your business. As much of this is educated guess work, what trends do you think will become important as time moves forward?

Scent Marketing – the Amazing Sell

In the world of marketing, businesses have essentially made use of every sensory avenue they could think of, from sight to sound to touch, to convince customers to buy their product or to create a positive brand image. One of the less travelled avenues that are gathering traffic today is the olfactory kind, and retailers all over the world are trying to find that perfect smell of success to boost their sales. However, the business of **scent marketing** is much more complex than that, as we will soon find out.

Why does scent work so well?

The fact that scent has been so under-used in the world of marketing is surprising, since the science of smell suggests it is probably more effective than all the other senses it employs. In simple terms, when we get a whiff of something, the smell is transmitted to and interpreted by the olfactory bulb which is part of the limbic system. This part of our brain is also responsible for memory and emotion, which means we link smell with pleasant or unpleasant experiences instantaneously, bringing subconscious levels of strong nostalgia. This is why we associate certain smells from the beach or a resort we stayed in with good times and pleasant vacation memories.

Our other senses such as sight, sound, taste, or touch can also trigger memories and emotion but not as instantaneously. This is due to the fact that they travel to the cognitive receptors of the brain and thus, we can apply some conscious reasoning to these. Since smell works on such a subconscious level, it is more effective in triggering an impulsive reaction from buyers.

This is the reason why more and more businesses are rushing towards scent as a way of branding and marketing their products. A story in Times Magazine reports predictions by a consulting firm based in New York, which states that expenditures on scent marketing spanned between $50m and $80m last year, and this number is anticipated to rise above $500m in the next 10 years.

Types of scent marketing

Scent marketing has different uses for different business, and so can be effectively divided into four distinct types. There is the Aroma Billboard Smell, which makes the boldest scent statement and is the most "there", that is, the customers are consciously aware of it, such as the trademark smell of freshly brewed coffee at Starbucks. The smell is part of the customer experience and it is what consciously attracts them.

On the other hand, a Thematic Smell complements the décor or purpose of the place, such as vanilla or lavender smells at a beauty spa or a resort. Ambient Smells are more subtle and create an atmosphere, used to cover unpleasant odors or to "fill a void". Lastly, a Signature Smell is exclusive to a big brand name and is used to create a brand image; customers associate this smell with their favourite brand and what it represents, such as the smells of cardamom and ivory used by the high-end shoe brand Jimmy Choo to emanate wealth and luxury.

Change Things Up in Your Business Demographic - The Benefits to Using Scent in Marketing

Scents can help boost sales

We've already discussed some of the benefits; it can trigger instant emotional reactions from customers. Scent marketing can thus be very effective in boosting sales. A study done by Nike discovered that they could increase the intent to purchase by 80% through the introduction of scent into their stores. Another survey at a petrol station with a mini-mart reported that the aroma of coffee helped boost sales of the beverage by a whopping 300%.

Scents make customers linger

Scents can also help customers linger in a store and look around more. Eric Spangenberg, the dean of the College of Business at Washington State University, was the first to look for scientific evidence of this in 1996 through a lab study in Pullman. He found subjects were more likely to look around and browse through products in the rooms that were scented, and reported more positive opinions and a tendency to wait longer in lines in the fake store than its unscented counterpart.

Scents help create brand image

Scents are helpful in making people remember you, or to create associations in their minds. This is why it can be useful it creating an all rounded brand image, such as the above Jimmy Choo example. Many hotels also use scents to make people associate them with good memories, such as the Westin Hotels' use of a blend of green tea, geranium and black cedar diffused into their lobbies, according to the New York Times' Key Magazine. The scent you use will obviously go with the image you want for your brand, whether it is luxury, comfort, quaint and old-fashioned or modern and contemporary.

Scents create a perception of quality

In general scents can also help create a perception of quality. Customers tend to perceive a scented product or space as being of better quality and will be willing to pay more when shopping in a scented store, as discovered by a study done by the Smell & Taste Research Foundation. Many of the subjects in the study reported that they were willing to pay 10$ more for Nike sneakers placed in scented rooms, than those placed in an unscented one.

The downside to using scents for marketing

On the other hand, scenting a space can also go horribly wrong. Using scent is much more tricky and complex than using music or visuals. A Wal-Mart in north Spokane had to be evacuated and one person even ended up in the hospital when an "unidentified odour" wafted out of the bathrooms and gave many shoppers headaches and dry mouth. Smells have the potential of creating unanticipated allergies in certain people, and in lesser degrees can cause people to simply leave a space, something unlikely to happen with, say, a bad song.

Scents can be highly subjective

Businesses must also deal with the subjective nature of smells, according to Spangenberg. This makes using smells highly risky and complex, especially when cultural appropriateness and gender come into play. Plus, scent works great when it is congruent with the business it is promoting, but if not done right, it can actually hurt the business more than when no scent is used. Spangenberg tested different smells to go with certain products. He saw that in a clothing store, floral scents only attracted women and fewer men, while masculine smells of rose maroc attracted more men and lesser women.

The kind of smell you use plays a huge role in the success of your campaign, Spangenberg suggests. His other studies show that people are more likely to respond to what they expect. The smells of holiday spices or chocolate chip cookies work better than ordinary, generic smells during

Christmas, for example. In another study he discovered that people are likely to spend 20% more in stores scented with simpler scents that they could instantly process rather than more complex smells.

How businesses can make use of it

With all this information in mind, many businesses have been able to make use of scents to sell their products more effectively. The key however, is to keep it natural, simple and diffuse, as overpowering and complex smells can be distracting and actually have negative effects. Also, as Spangenberg discovered, the scent you use should take into account your product and the gender, age, geography and culture of the target market. This is why many businesses go to scent marketing consultants to develop a scent marketing strategy with a customized and unique scent that would work for their business.

If we take the example of Cinnabon, we all love the smell of freshly baked Cinnabon, and this is always enticing for anyone who loves cinnamon rolls. However, this is no accident, but an entire strategy according to the President of Cinnabon, Kat Cole. The ovens are specifically placed at the front of the store the smell would waft out and spread throughout the malls and airports where the stores are usually located. The ventilations systems and oven covers used are also deliberately of lower quality, to help trap the sweet aromas in. Over here this successful chain utilizes natural odours to draw in their customers and boost sales.

On the other hand, a similar business where food smells are used, artificial smells are created. The M&M World store in Leicester Square, London stores pre-packaged goodies, and so utilized the services of a scent marketing company to create a chocolate aroma diffused around the store.

Other companies may use various artificial smells in line with their brand image and products, as we saw in the Jimmy Choo and Westin Hotels examples, or just as an ambient smell to create a pleasant atmosphere. This is usually done by vaporizing the scent through "nebulisation technology" using high-voltage, low current electricity. The dry vapour is then spread through the ventilation systems. I also know of one company in Australia that markets scent marketing using a battery powered automatic dispenser utilizing a very fine mist. This helps make the smell very subtle, working on a subconscious level and sort of becoming part of the environment instead of being consciously there.

CHAPTER 21: UNDERSTANDING AND APPRECIATING THE CUSTOMER

Social Media Customer Service

Everyone uses some form of social media and it is therefore natural that your customers would seek customer service from you on the social media platform they are most familiar with. In my experience it's an awful lot quicker and easier than picking up the telephone and waiting in a list to get to speak to someone. When you think about it, customer service isn't just about responding to negative complaints, requests for help, etc., it's also about servicing your customers by engaging with them when they're talking about your brand.

Social media allows you to listen to your customers and monitor issues before they even become a real problem. If you provide top-notch service, in a speedy manner you're going to increase customer loyalty in ways you may have never thought possible. It doesn't matter if you're a large corporation and well-known brand, or if you're a small bricks and mortar shop, or a sole proprietor running their business solely on the internet. Social media customer service demand is growing and it's here to stay, and it's time to find out how you can utilize it.

If you think about it, in the past unless a customer called with a complaint, the business had no idea anything was wrong. Today, with social media even if a customer doesn't contact you with an issue, they will talk about it and discuss it, on social media. It's up to you to listen, respond, and make it right. Social media platforms are where your customer are talking about you for bad and for good.

Good Customer Service Is the Best Marketing

The trouble with social media however is that it's possible to miss complaints which have been buried in other comments, but if you make it your business to read every single comment, not only might you find opportunities to provide excellent social media customer service by helping a customer or potential customer answer questions and fix problems, but you can also use the information gathered as a way to create new products and services for your market.

It's also a great idea create specific customer service social media accounts, and charge someone with the responsibility of keeping up with that account/s. If you choose this method, you'll need to remember to direct people in your other social media accounts to your customer service accounts. And remember you might still miss issues if there are people who don't pay attention and go to the right account so you'll still need to monitor all social media accounts. For a small business that rarely receives complaints, this can seem like a little much and to be honest you are missing a trick as solving customer complains helps new customers make purchasing decisions, because they know you are there supporting people.

You can also create a new Tab on Facebook that links customers to your customer service ticketing system, FAQ or knowledge base to make it easy for customers who connect with you on social media to resolve issues. Keep in mind that even with these additions you're still going to need to be actively engaged with your social media pages to ensure that all issues are handled quickly, responsibly and positively.

Customer Experience as a Story

One of the best ways to think about the customer experience is as a story, this is how your customers experiences it. The story starts with their first contact with your business, whether directly or indirectly. The plot thickens as they learn about your products or services and as they begin interacting with you.

The plot takes a major step forward when the customer decides to buy something from you, and the story continues as the customer's relationship with your business moves forward to future purchases and interactions.

Why It's Useful to Think of the Customer Experience as a Story

When we're evaluating the efficiency of our methods, we tend to look at data. This data can come to us in the form of statistics like sales data or web analytics, or from customers themselves in the form of survey results. But this data can't fully convey the customer experience as the customer experiences it.

This data isn't useful because it doesn't convey the totality of the customer experience, and that's exactly what it is, a totality. Rather, this data gives you only the specific data it can, such as how much web traffic you're getting or whether or not your customers think your response time is fast enough. If you're lucky, you'll get a few sentences of feedback, but even this isn't enough.

The customer experiences their journey with your business as a story, like any good movie or novel, each scene plays a part in the overall story. In order to understand what's working well or what's going wrong with your customer experience, you need to know the entire story and how all of the small parts fit together.

Know Your Customer's Story

The best way to learn your customer's story with your business is to put yourself in your customer's shoes and write out this story. You do this through mapping the customer experience. A customer experience map starts with the first contact you have with your customer and works its way through all of the story's "scenes," which are the individual touch points you have with the customer.

A customer experience map is something like an infographic which shows the entire story. With this you can take in the big picture at a glance, but it also shows you all of the relationships between the different parts. You can more easily see where problems might occur and areas where you can make improvements in order to maximize the experience.

There are many different ways to approach mapping the **customer experience**, but it should always be in story form. You should understand your business's customer experience through the customer's eyes.

CHAPTER 22: CLOSING THOUGHTS

Now that you've had an opportunity to read the entire formula and gain some fantastic ideas on how to become a millionaire as an entrepreneur in your field, the book ultimately has to come to an end.

Many people will make the grave mistake of putting this book down and never implementing the full spectrum of ideas available to them. Don't be one of those people. Put everything available to you income-wise into play. Become the millionaire I know you can be. You have potential!

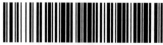

Made in the USA
San Bernardino, CA
15 February 2018